Profiles and Portfolios

Profiles and Portfolios

A guide for nurses and midwives

Cathy Hull and Liz Redfern

MACMILLAN

First published 1996 by
MACMILLAN PRESS LTD
Houndmills, Basingstoke, Hampshire RG21 6XS
and London
Companies and representatives
throughout the world

ISBN 0–333–60684–1

A catalogue record for this book is available
from the British Library.

10	9	8	7	6	5	4	3	2	1
05	04	03	02	01	00	99	98	97	96

Printed and bound in Great Britain by T. J. Press (Padstow) Ltd.

This book is dedicated to Vernon, Tiny and Mike, for being there and for their encouragement all along the way.

Contents

Foreword

Almost every nurse practising today will have attended, at one time or another, an award ceremony where 'the great and the good' will have taken a leaf out of Winston Churchill's book and reminded them – albeit in a different context – that 'this is not the end . . . it is the end of the beginning'. This advice has always been accompanied by the speaker stressing the need for the newly qualified practitioner to continue to learn to develop the newly acquired skills, knowledge and competences so that they can continue to provide a high standard of safe patient care.

Over the decades since I was at such a ceremony, such continuing professional development has become much easier and much more attractive. The 1970s saw the introduction and establishment of such bodies as The Joint Board of Clinical Nursing Studies (JBCNS), which offered combined clinical and education programmes in a wide range of specialist areas and of varying depth and length. By the late 1970s, the Diploma and Degree programmes were established. Such programmes as the University of London Diploma (which became a degree course in the 1980s) brought part-time advanced study to those nurses who could not reach a fixed study site such as a conventional College or University.

By the 1980s, we had integrated programmes developing, offering academic and professional credits, and the early 1990s found an even wider menu available, as the Open University and Open College joined the provider market.

The authors of the book grew up as I did, with these changes. Even more importantly, both were, and still are, actively involved in the field of published Open Learning, such as the *Nursing Times* programmes, the DLC (Distance Learning Centre) Projects and Health Pickup.

As the profession demanded a more flexible and accessible

xi

approach to continuing professional education, the National Boards and the UKCC moved to validate the opportunities and to approve the innovative programmes developing within the (then) Schools of Nursing and their associated Universities.

But many staff had qualifications which had been gained before such validations. Many more had attended the conferences, study days and workshops which were increasingly being offered, and nurses were also realising that there were things they did, other than nursing, which had merit. Examples included voluntary work and youth work.

So we saw the development of APL and APEL (Accreditation of Prior [Experiential] Learning). Again, the authors were involved in this initiative.

In order to support so much learning, so many opportunities, the profession was supported by mentors, preceptors, supervisors . . .

Nurses everywhere have been inundated with advice about not only what to do and how to do it, but what to do with it when you've done it. The profession has been swamped with information on reflective practice, validation, accreditation, profiling, portfolio, APL, APEL, CATS (Credit Accumulation Transfer Scheme), CAL (Computer Assisted Learning), CEPS (Continuing Education Points scheme) and all the other educational and practice development jargon.

Confused? Join the crowd!

But two people who aren't confused are Cathy Hull and Liz Redfern. They have been amongst the leaders in Professional Development for many years and are most ably equipped to guide any nurse through the labyrinth of developing and maintaining the professional portfolio we all need. They debunk the myths, explain the terms, clarify what you need to do and – perhaps more importantly – what you do not need to do, and offer clear advice on the many ways nurses can fulfil their own continuing education needs to maintain competence and meet the requirements of PREP (Post-Registration Education for Practice). They answer every question you've thought of, as well as many you haven't. In short, to go back to Winston Churchill – they have indeed 'give[n] us the tools' we all need to understand the complex work of continuing professional development and the development and maintenance of our profiles and portfolios.

Dr Betty Kershaw

Acknowledgements

We would like to acknowledge Linda Davidson for bringing us together to speak about profiles at the first Nursing Times Staff Nurse conference in Scarborough in 1992. The conference venue was the Spa and the opening session was held in what looked like an old music hall theatre with lights all around the stage. We had never met before, but we knew then that we shared the same sense of humour, passion and values about how people learn and develop.

This book would not have been possible unless we had had the opportunity to share, discuss and develop our ideas and understanding with a whole range of people along the way. The entire list would fill the book; however, we would like to thank the following for their generosity of spirit, encouragement, knowledge and time:

Susan Fey
Sue Frost
Rob Imeson
Chris James
Chris Johns
Jan Kelly

Marianne Phillips
Jill Rogers
John Storan
Claire Virgo
Susan Weil
Debra Witmer

Special thanks to Michelle Murtagh for helping with the typing, Jan Kelly for compiling the bibliography, and Debra Witmer and Maggie Wallace for their contributions and support.

Introduction

The idea for developing this book came from our experience of speaking at nursing conferences and running workshops, and our direct involvement in helping people understand and put together profiles in a nursing and midwifery context.

Our experience led us to realise that although people quickly grasp the idea that profiling can help them to develop, they then do not know how to start. They are unsure of the practical issues, such as how to develop a profile and how they can relate it to their practice. The common questions asked in workshops are:

- Do I need to buy one?
- If I do, which one is likely to meet my needs?
- Can I do one on my own or do I need help?
- How do I express my life experience in a containable, meaningful way?
- Where do I start?

The aim of this book is to give people practical guidance on the whole continuum of profile work, from start to completion, accepting that it can be a never-ending process. The book is based on what we think people need to know to make a success of profiling and, more importantly, the issues people commonly ask for help with.

This book will give people guidance in compiling their own profiles. It is intended to act in support of the process, rather than to provide a model profile. Although we suggest activities and include an annotated bibliography of resource material that will help with the process, this is not a book that you work through, using activities to create a profile. It is intended to support the whole process of profiling.

Readers will bring their own styles and learning needs to the book and should use it in a way that works for them. We have written it knowing that most readers will dip in and out when they have particular learning needs, rather than read it sequentially. Each chapter has an introductory section which will help people decide if that chapter is relevant. However, the chapters do follow a logical sequence and order, which will help readers who want to read from cover to cover. It would be almost impossible to write a book that covers all the specific needs for specific educational programmes, so we have not tried to do this.

Readers will be aware that the terms profile and portfolio are used interchangeably in nursing and midwifery. This issue is addressed in several chapters and we will not repeat the arguments here. We have decided to use the term profile throughout the book unless referring to a specific product called a portfolio, because Personal Professional Profile is the term that has been chosen by the UKCC.

The book gave the opportunity for two people to combine their experience of profiles from different backgrounds for the benefits of the reader. Cathy Hull has a background in adult education, experiential processes and facilitating others in the profile process from outside nursing. Liz Redfern brings her experience of profiles and reflective practice from a professional context of nursing and midwifery practice and education. Both of us believe that as individuals we could not have written the same book, and its quality has been considerably enhanced by our collaboration. We hope you enjoy the book as much as we enjoyed working together writing it.

So what does the book contain? The following chapter-by-chapter breakdown gives an overview.

Chapter 1 Profiles and Portfolios: The Nursing and Midwifery Context

This chapter charts the history and identifies the factors, such as the statutory bodies, reflective practice, market forces and higher education, that have influenced the introduction of profiles into nursing and midwifery. It also contains the outline of a profile initiative in Ontario.

Chapter 2   Getting to Grips with the Terminology

This chapter attempts to unravel the confusion in the terminology so that everyone can understand it and use it appropriately.

Chapter 3   Some Common Themes and Questions Shared

Here we explore the ten most common questions asked about profiles.

Chapter 4   Getting Started: Creating Your Personal Profile

In this chapter you will find practical advice and activities on how to develop a framework for your profile.

Chapter 5   Profiles and Reflective Practice

This chapter attempts to demystify the concept of reflective practice and offers some practical strategies for beginners.

Chapter 6   Making Your Learning Count

This chapter will be helpful for those who are developing a profile specifically to seek accreditation within an educational programme or system.

Chapter 7   Helping Others to Develop a Profile: The Skills of Facilitation

In this chapter we look at some of the specific skills and knowledge you will need to help someone else to complete a profile. We look at how adults learn and explore the five key skills of facilitation. This chapter is written with practitioners in mind, but it might also be useful for teachers.

Epilogue

This concluding chapter includes the transcript of a conversation between the two authors. It is their contribution to the continuing debate on profiling.

Annotated Bibliography

We realised that it would be helpful for readers to have access to resources that will help them with the profiling process. The resource material which has been annotated in this chapter comes from several disciplines.

Profiles and Portfolios: The Nursing and Midwifery Context

1

This chapter charts the history and identifies the factors, such as the statutory bodies, reflective practice, market forces and higher education, that have influenced the introduction of profiles into the nursing and midwifery world. It goes on to explore the way profiles are being commonly used at present and addresses such issues as confidentiality. The final part of the chapter outlines an initiative in Ontario, Canada, to introduce profiles as part of a quality assurance programme.

The use of a personal profile is now a statutory requirement for all nurses, midwives and health visitors wishing to remain on the register. The decision of the United Kingdom Council for Nursing, Midwifery and Health Visiting (UKCC) to bring in this type of legislation means that profiles are not a passing trend. This opening chapter sets the scene by identifying the factors that have influenced the groundswell of profile activity in nursing and midwifery. Whilst the UKCC requirement means that everyone on the register will have to maintain a Personal Professional Profile in accordance with guidelines, there are a lot of other reasons for maintaining a profile. We hope this book will help you to understand them in the widest possible context.

Influences on the development of profiles and portfolios

Articles about the use of profiles and portfolios began to appear in British nursing and midwifery literature in 1993. However, like most major changes in professional behaviour, it is difficult to pinpoint exactly when or who started the ball rolling. Factors such as the statutory bodies, reflective practice, market forces and higher education have all influenced their development.

Statutory bodies

Statutory bodies have been influential in introducing the concept of profiles and portfolios, and they continue to support their use. This is interesting, as it is more usual for the statutory bodies to appear to lag behind the profession in educational development, because of their necessarily slow decision-making processes. In this instance, however, we have the statutory bodies firmly in the lead – making the use of a Personal Professional Profile a statutory requirement.

Since April 1995, the UKCC has *required* individuals on the professional register to use a Personal Professional Profile. The use of a profile will be part of the UKCC's requirement for maintaining effective registration. In effect, the requirement will be introduced over a period of time and everyone must be using a profile by the *next* time they renew their registration in three years' time. That is, if you wish to re-register every three years, you will need to show how you have been maintaining professional knowledge and competence by meeting the UKCC's requirements for the equivalent of a minimum of five days' updating. The UKCC expects this continuing education activity to be recorded in your Personal Professional Profile, along with a summary of your key personal and professional details.

These requirements are outcomes of the PREP report. In March 1994, the UKCC issued a paper, *The Future of Professional Practice: The Council's Standards for Education and*

Practice Following Registration. This document was essentially the final chapter of the PREP report, which had started life in the late 1980s. In the paper, the UKCC explains its approach to profiles and says this has been chosen 'to help practitioners identify their personal and practice related study needs and then to choose the relevant activity to meet such needs'.

In the same month as making this statement, the UKCC announced it would not be issuing everyone on the register with a 'free' profile. Instead, the UKCC undertook to provide everyone with guidelines about all aspects of PREP, including personal profiles. These were made available as a series of fact sheets to all registrants during Spring 1995.

Two of the National Boards in the UK have also played a part in influencing and increasing professional awareness about the use of profiles and portfolios.

The Welsh National Board (WNB) was the first to produce a Professional Profile Folder. It became available in 1991 at the time that the use of personal organisers was becoming more widespread, and it uses that design approach. The layout related to the then newly launched WNB continuing education framework at diploma level, but the general principles used to design the profile could also be applied by practitioners not following the WNB framework.

The English National Board (ENB) then produced its framework for continuing professional education. This framework is designed around ten key characteristics of professional practice, which are said to represent the benchmarks of expert professional practice They are about:

1 professional accountability and responsibility
2 clinical expertise with a specific client group
3 use of research to plan, implement and evaluate strategies to improve care
4 team working and building, and multi-disciplinary team leadership
5 flexible and innovative approaches to care
6 use of health promotion strategies
7 facilitating and assessing development in others

8   handling information and making informed clinical decisions
9   setting standards and evaluating quality of care
10 initiating, managing and evaluating clinical change.

There are two ways to use the framework. Firstly, the overall structure of the ten key characteristics can be used to plan your individual professional development. Secondly, the framework can be used as a way to construct a modular programme, which is validated by a university to give an honours degree and by the ENB to give the Higher Award.

A key component of the ENB framework, whichever way it is being used, is the Professional Portfolio. This was first published in November 1991 and was revised and reissued in 1995. The use of the portfolio is compulsory for those who are indexed with the ENB for the Higher Award. The ENB also promotes its portfolio as a useful professional development tool which will be helpful to everyone. Its popularity is demonstrated by the fact that sales far exceed the number of practitioners indexed with the ENB for the Higher Award.

The recognition by the statutory bodies about how profiles and portfolios can be used by professionals is important. It gives profiles and portfolios a strong standing within the profession which could not have been achieved so quickly had the statutory bodies not been involved. The fact that personal profiles will be part of the legislative process involved in the implementation of PREP also ensures they are not a passing phase.

Terminology

Some readers may be wondering about our apparent inconsistent use of terminology. We have, however, used the terminology correctly, as applied by the different statutory bodies. For example, the ENB calls its product a Professional Portfolio, whilst the UKCC talks about a Personal Professional Profile. In our experience, the terms profile and portfolio are used interchangeably and often inaccurately. Chapter 2 discusses the terminology associated with profiles and portfolios in some detail. At this point the terminology is not important, except to note that within nursing and midwifery there appears to be some confusion and inconsistency. From now on we will use the term profile, unless talking about a specific product which calls itself a portfolio.

Reflective practice

A parallel development in nursing and midwifery has been the rise in popularity of reflective practice. We go into reflective practice in more detail in Chapter 5 and it is discussed here in the context of its supporting influence on profiles.

Any readers who have recently completed a course or programme at a pre-registration or post-registration level are likely to have been asked to complete a reflective journal or diary. The majority of commercially available profiles encourage their owners to reflect and to use them as a storage place for the outcomes of the reflective process. Some also give guidance on the art of reflection.

During 1994 the ENB reviewed its portfolio with several Higher Award approved centres. One of the criticisms was that, whilst encouraging reflective practice, there was in-sufficient guidance about what was involved in reflective practice and how to go about it. The ENB responded to this criticism by issuing an additional guidance booklet with its portfolio – one section of the booklet addresses reflective practice in more depth.

By encouraging reflective practice, profiles generate further interest in reflective practice; and, in a reciprocal way, reflective practitioners need to write about their reflections and a profile is a useful place to do this. However, it would be unrealistic to expect a profile to be totally self-contained, and it will always be necessary to supplement any guidance it might give by further reading on the subject of reflection and reflective practice. Chapter 5 is a good place to start.

There is often professional concern expressed about how confidential and secure a record of reflective practice within a profile can be. Once you have committed the outcomes of your reflection to paper or computer disk, who does it belong to? Who has the right to see it? There have been some occasions when the contents of personal diaries or reflective journals have been subpoenaed as evidence within cases of professional conduct or litigation. Confidentiality is an ongoing issue which has yet to be satisfactorily resolved. We are aware that the UKCC is continuing to seek legal advice on this issue and guidance is likely to be available in the future. Of course, you need to remember that, were you called to give evidence in such a case, you would be expected to 'tell the truth and nothing but the whole truth' as a law-abiding citizen, and a reflective journal may be useful in jogging your memory. Just because you decide not to write it down in your profile does not mean an occurrence or incident did not happen, and you would be expected to give the details of it as verbal evidence if asked to do so. The writings in the reflective section of a profile merely bring your memory of events into sharper focus.

Putting the potential spectre of giving evidence aside for a moment, under normal circumstances you have a choice about what to record, and a further point of choice about what you share and when and with whom you share it. The issue of confidentiality is addressed in more detail in Chapter 5.

We believe the outcomes of reflective practice and the learning that occurs is nursing and midwifery knowledge in the making. In the past nurses and midwives relied on the information found in text books and articles to help them know what to do and when. But this knowledge can also be developed through the insights gained during reflective practice, which has the benefit of being grounded in practice. Perhaps the nursing and midwifery text books of the future will be comprised of extracts from the profiles of reflective practitioners.

Adult and higher education

Nursing and midwifery have a relatively short history of using profiles. They have been introduced primarily as a professional development tool within a continuing education context, and their introduction has been heavily influenced by educationalists. Educationalists in nursing and midwifery have, in recent years, received their preparation as teachers within the wider context of adult and higher education. This has made them aware of the ways profiles are being used within alternative contexts to nursing and health care:

- a profile approach to assessment
- as part of a claim for prior learning within a credit accumulation and transfer scheme
- the use of learning contracts within profiles
- the student-centred approach which profiles encourage.

The open learning approach which a profile offers to the student is also attractive to many nursing and midwifery teachers, because it gives them the role of facilitator rather than teacher. We discuss facilitation skills in more detail in Chapter 7.

Market forces

As soon as it became obvious that maintaining a Personal Professional Profile would become a statutory requirement for all those on the register, several publishing houses extended their interest beyond text books and journals for nurses and midwives and into producing profiles. The potential market for selling these commercially produced profiles is large and it became open to all once the UKCC announced they would not be producing their own to give 'free' to all registrants. The profiles available for purchase vary tremendously with respect to quality and the approach taken. In most instances, the one you decide to buy will depend as much on personal preference as anything else. If you have not already purchased a profile for personal use, then this book should help you understand more about why and how you might use one, and therefore enable you to judge which one will suit your personal needs. There is more information in Chapter 3 on this subject.

Some of the products for sale are no more than ring binders with dividers and a place to record personal and professional details. Others take you deeply into the realms of self-awareness. Yet more are linked to specific continuing professional development programmes and are as much educationally driven as commercially driven. The *Profile Pack*, which originated as part of the Nursing Times Open Learning (NTOL) initiative (now Macmillan Open Learning), is a good example of a profile which is driven educationally within a commercial context.

The widespread awareness that exists within the profession could not have been achieved by the statutory bodies alone. The power of the marketing and advertising strategies of the publishing houses has made a major contribution to heightening awareness, however superficial, of the existence of profiles.

The rise in popularity in profiles has also inspired many colleges of nursing and midwifery to produce their own. It is now quite common to find colleges selling a profile designed to complement the corporate image of the college.

Many nurses ask whether it will be sufficient to compile their own profile using a ring binder. Do you really need to buy a ready-made product? The UKCC (Fact Sheet 4) gives the following advice:

> You may choose one of the many profiles now available through various bodies such as professional organisations, publishers and some of the four National Boards for Nursing, Midwifery and Health Visiting in the UK. Alternatively, you may decide to create your own profile document simply using a ring binder.

The only point that we would like to add is that most of the ready-made profiles have been developed by experts and have been field tested. The resources put into that activity should be of benefit to you, the user, and should give you confidence in the way you use the profile.

One of the criticisms of ready-made profiles is that they look too smart. Nurses and midwives often say they are apprehensive about writing in them for fear of making them look untidy. It is true that many users prefer to keep their bought profile for a special occasion, such as a job interview or some final presentation of their work. It will be necessary to use a lot of supplementary note books or files to keep all the information and observations you will acquire over the period of your professional life. Anyone who practises reflection is likely to want to have a pocket-sized note book to make jot ings during the working day. Such a note book is likely to become dog-eared and its contents will need to be reviewed from time to time. The review will enable decisions to be made about what needs to be transferred into a more permanent file.

Uses within nursing and midwifery

There will be lots of reasons why readers will pick up this book. It may be that you want to know more about the subject generally, or you may have been prompted to find out more for a specific purpose.

Profiles are currently used mainly within a continuing education context, because, as previously mentioned, the impetus has come from the PREP debate and legislation. In time, it is likely that all pre-registration students will gain exposure to and experience in the use of profiles – they will become an integral part of professional behaviour. Many schools also use the profile concept and so people entering nursing will already be familiar with the approach. In the meantime, most nurses and midwives start using profiles for a particular reason and then broaden their use over time. The ENB guidelines (1995) on using their portfolio suggest it can be used as:

- a record of professional experience, therefore contributing to meeting the PREP requirements
- part of the process of applying for a job
- part of an individual performance review (IPR) process, by helping you to identify personal goals and how these are to be achieved

- a focus for organising your own learning
- a way to support learning from practice and clinical supervision
- a tool for reflective practice
- a means of achieving accreditation as part of a prior learning claim
- a way of demonstrating learning for assessment towards the ENB Higher Award (or other educational programmes).

This is a fairly comprehensive list and covers most of the ways in which profiles are currently being used in nursing and midwifery.

PREP requirements

We have already discussed the UKCC's requirements for individuals to maintain a Personal Professional Profile as part of the PREP legislation. The detail of what the UKCC expect is clearly outlined in their Fact Sheet 4, entitled *Your Personal Professional Profile*. If you would like a fact sheet, contact the UKCC at 23 Portland Place, London W1N 4JT.

Job applications

It is now common, particularly when applying for a more senior post, to be asked for a curriculum vitae (CV) to accompany or replace the traditional job application forms. It is certainly easier to construct a CV using information extracted from a well-maintained profile than from your memory or elusive bits of paper kept in a safe place. Nurses and midwives have been known to take their whole profile to the job interview. It is always worth checking in advance if this amount of information is expected or needed. More usually prospective employers expect you to pick out those experiences from your past career that have a particular bearing on your current job application.

Identifying personal goals

Most grades of staff now experience a form of performance review on a periodic basis. Each employer will have a different scheme for assessing and reviewing performance. Most schemes include an opportunity for you to look back on the previous year and identify achievements and disappointments. They also have a section where you are asked to look forward to the forthcoming year and identify what personal development needs you might have to enable you to fulfil your role.

The looking back and thinking forward can be much easier if you have maintained a profile, as it is likely to contain details of formal or informal learning opportunities you have had during the year. Reflection on critical incidents will identify areas where you feel particularly confident and areas where you need further training or experience. All this information can be very useful when completing a self-assessment exercise as part of the performance review paperwork.

Focus for organising your own learning

When you are enrolled on a particular course or programme of study, it is easier to organise your learning agenda around the demands of the course. This is not always the case when you are working hard and have no particular focus for your learning and no impetus for writing about the learning. A profile can therefore provide a focus for learning, in a number of ways:

- a storehouse for relevant articles and references
- a place where you can write notes, on a regular basis, about what you have learnt and what you need to find out more about
- a place where you can record the outcomes of any self-assessment and what you would need to do to act on these.

Using a profile in this way means you have to discipline yourself to review the contents on a regular basis. This review helps you to make sense of the contents – to see where you have been, say, over the past three months. Looking back on a range of experiences in this way can be a useful springboard to knowing what needs to happen next on your learning pathway. It can also be a great confidence booster, as it helps you realise how much you have achieved and what you are capable of.

Supporting learning from practice and clinical supervision

The points to be made here are very similar to those made above. One of the most effective ways of learning from your practice is to write about it. You will often find that, in the act of writing about something you did, you will get deeper insights into the subject. These insights are, more often than not, associated with points of *real* learning about the way that you practise. Nurses and midwives who practise clinical supervision often spend time writing up the process in their profile, if they have one. It is so easy to realise something in a clinical supervision session, only to forget it again in the busy activity of nursing or midwifery. Writing about it gives it a greater chance of being committed to memory, and therefore a greater chance of being remembered and practised the next time you come across that situation.

Tool for reflective practice

Reflective practice has already been mentioned in this chapter and will be explored in more detail in Chapter 5.

Achieving accreditation as part of a prior learning claim

The concept of gaining credit for prior learning is relatively new in nursing and midwifery, although it has been available in higher education for some time. It gained particular support and impetus with the publication of the government White Paper *Higher Education: Meeting the Challenge* (1987).

The ENB legitimised accreditation for prior learning (APL) and accreditation for prior experiential learning (APEL) in nursing and midwifery post-registration programmes when it launched its framework for continuing professional education in 1991. The ENB insisted that the mechanisms for assessing prior learning had to be available for those indexing for the Higher Award. The ENB *Professional Portfolio,* which was issued at the same time, was intended to be helpful to those who wished to compile evidence for a prior learning claim.

Using the contents of a profile or portfolio in this way needs careful guidance and the ability to discriminate what is relevant to the claim and what to leave out. Nurses and midwives often assume that getting credit for prior learning will be far easier than attending the course. This is not the case – we look at the process of applying for credit in detail in Chapter 6, to give you a realistic view of what is involved.

Assessment for an educational programme

You may be asked to submit sections of your profile as part of an assessment scheme for a course or programme you are following. In these circumstances you need to be quite clear what is expected of you and the confidentiality of the information you are handing in. The confidentiality section of Chapter 5 gives you more information on this.

Life-long learning

Profiles are part of a model of learning which is being adopted by an increasing number of health care educators. This new model about developing life-long learners 'looks to the nature of learning, rather than the methods of instruction' (Ferguson, 1981). It is now more important than ever in the rapidly changing world of health that any form of education for health care professionals should foster the capacity to go on learning. Health service employers now demand and expect employees to be flexible, self-motivated and able to transfer skills into new situations with ease. In addition, they need to be able to demonstrate problem-solving abilities and decision-making skills. This all needs personal confidence and, of course, it requires practitioners to be up to date. At the same time, funds and available time for attending formal courses are being reduced, so you need to be able to learn effectively from your own experience.

The skills involved in developing and maintaining your own profile are skills that will help you develop as a life-long learner.

An international perspective: profiles in nursing in Ontario

The majority of this chapter has been devoted to the UK nursing and midwifery context – rightly so as we are still trying to grasp the implications of introducing profiles in the UK for these professions. However, we are not the only nursing community that is being challenged by using profiles. This section describes initiatives being implemented by the Colleges of Nursing of Ontario (CNO). Their motives were not dissimilar to those of the UKCC, and you will see from the events and actions described below how influential the UK approach to profiles has been in shaping the Ontario experience. We are grateful to Debra Witmer of the CNO for providing the material for this section of the chapter. We felt it was important to give the book an international perspective and our contact with Debra during her period of researching the UK profiling scene gave us an ideal opportunity.

The CNO is the governing body for 150 000 registered nurses and registered practical nurses in the province of Ontario (Canada). It had to find a way of responding to a new Ontario Government Act which became law in 1991. The Regulated Health Professions Act, 1991, was passed partially in response to an increasing pressure for greater professional accountability to the public. In anticipation of the Act, the CNO began to develop a new quality assurance programme which was multi-faceted and comprehensive. It contained two components: quality control and quality improvement. The quality control element focused on establishing and enforcing baseline standards. Quality improvement focused on the competence of individual members as well as data gathering, to provide continuous feedback on programme evaluation, the settings within which members practise, and the profession as a whole.

There was a growing discontent with the effectiveness of mandatory programmes that require a number of course credits, hours of instruction, and periodic general testing. This discontent helped set the stage for a facilitative rather than punitive approach to competence assurance. The CNO believe that the maintenance and improvement of competence cannot be dictated, but must come from the practitioner's own sense of accountability and responsibility. This is in keeping with the principles underlying adult education and professional development. These beliefs have led to a programme being developed that promotes accountability and responsibility through self-assessment, learning associates or peer assessment; identification of learning needs from practice experience; and continuous learning through the creation of learning projects designed and implemented by the individual practitioner. These approaches lend themselves comfortably to the use of a profile.

While mandatory programmes place accountability and responsibility for the identification of learning needs and learning solutions on the regulatory body, the Professional Profile Portfolio being introduced by the CNO places the responsibility in the hands of the individual professional. In this way, maintaining and improving competence is integrated and becomes a 'state of mind' for the individual. The regulatory body is therefore able to focus on support and assistance. The CNO believe that this approach is the most appropriate way to ensure the ongoing maintenance and improvement of competence, and therefore the best mechanism for protecting the public interest.

One of the most exciting aspects of the programme focuses on the use of a Professional Profile Portfolio. The CNO researched the PREP initiatives in the UK when developing their own profile.

The CNO's use of a profile specifically to assess and assure the continuing competence of nursing is a first for North America and is breaking new ground and providing leadership for other regulatory bodies in that part of the world. Profiles are being used in the USA and other parts of Canada, but are primarily designed to assess life- and work-related experience with a view to obtaining academic credit. They are mainly used within academic institutions.

The CNO Professional Profile Portfolio is composed of a manual and a workbook and includes a core profile, a standards-based self-assessment tool, and a learning plan. It provides a positive approach to promoting continuing competence through reflective self-assessment. The core profile is designed to lead members, by the use of specific reflective exercises, through an assessment of their professional, educational and personal experiences. This process not only provides members with a context for understanding the course of their professional development, but also assists them in developing a clear understanding of their own particular learning style – which in turn helps them to learn more effectively.

The profile provides nurses with a framework for identifying and reflecting on their experience, so they know what they have learnt and what they need to learn. They begin by identifying past personal experiences that were significant because they marked or stimulated change, or were simply memorable. They then reflect on these activities in order to identify what they learnt and how the events affected them personally or professionally. Because the reflective exercises are based on each individual's practices, the outcomes are directly relevant to the profile user. The goal is for nurses to be able to plan their learning so that it relates to their practice and then to choose educational activities that are accessible and relevant.

The CNO are planning a range of support activities to help members fulfil the requirements of the quality assurance programme and the profile. The profile concept reflects the philosophy of the quality assurance programme being developed and represents a new mind-set toward the regulations of professionals. The programme seeks to protect public interest through the promotion of self-assessment and reflection, with the goal of continuing competence through individualised continuous learning. This goal is similar to the life-long learning approach that we have already discussed.

References

ENB (1991) *ENB Framework for Continuing Professional Education for Nurses, Midwives and Health Visitors: Guide to Implementation*, ENB Publications: London

Department of Education (1987) *Higher Education: Meeting the Challenge*, HMSO: London.

ENB (1994) *Using Your Portfolio: A Resource for Practitioners*, ENB Publications: London

Macmillan Open Learning (1994) *Profile Pack*, Macmillan Magazines: London

UKCC (1994) *The Future of Professional Practice: The Council's Standards for Education and Practice Following Registration*, UKCC: London.

UKCC (1995) *Fact Sheet 4: Your Personal Professional Profile*, UKCC: London

Ferguson, M. (1981) *The Aquarian Conspiracy: Personal and Social Transformation in the 1980s*, Paladin: London

Getting to Grips with the Terminology 2

The introduction of the profile has brought with it a new range of jargon that is unfamiliar and at times confusing. To make matters worse, the terms profile and portfolio are often used interchangeably and sometimes inaccurately. This chapter attempts to explain the terminology and unravel the jargon by clarifying the following terms: continuing professional development, life-long learning, profile, portfolio, experiential learning, reflection, CATS, APL, APEL and learning outcomes.

The introduction of profiles into the world of nursing and midwifery has brought with it new terms and jargon with which readers may not be familiar. Many of them come from the context of adult and higher education, and, whilst not difficult to understand in themselves, they are strange and unfamiliar. However, if nurses and midwives are to gain the benefits that can come from using a profile, they must get to grips with the terms used. This chapter will help you understand the distinctions and meanings behind some of the key terms associated with profiles. It should help you understand what people are talking about when they use the terms and enable you to use them accurately within your own professional language. All the terms described here will also be considered in more depth in the other chapters.

Continuing professional development and life-long learning

No nurse or midwife could have failed to notice that there is pressure to continue to develop as a professional after completion of an initial registration course. There are many reasons why nurses and midwives need continuing professional development. The first is that they need to keep up to date with new developments in knowledge, under-standing, technical skills and procedures. Just as the professions are constantly changing, so also professionals need to be able to adapt to the changes and to prepare themselves for the additional roles which will be demanded of them. Health care professionals need to become far more self-aware, reflective practitioners.

The rapidly changing scene of today's health service needs staff who are adaptable, flexible and able to expand their expertise and practice in response to what is happening around them. The current jargon for this approach is 'life-long learning'. This does not only mean coming to grips with a new knowledge base because of some new type of medical treatment that is now available; it also includes under-standing the skills you possess and how they can be quickly transferred from one situation to another. The ENB (1994) recently described life-long learners as being:

- **innovative** in their practice
- **flexible** to changing demand
- **resourceful** in their methods of working
- able to work as **change agents**
- able to **share good practice** and knowledge
- **adaptable** to changing health care needs
- challenging and **creative** in their practice
- **self-reliant** in their way of working
- **responsible and accountable** for their work.

We would want to add to this list 'someone who can use a profile approach to learning'. This is because in today's health service, which is under tremendous pressure, it is extremely likely that you will be expected to achieve these characteristics through your own learning initiative and not from attending a continuing education programme.

To continue to develop as a professional you also have to develop as a person. Although personal and professional development are sometimes expressed as separate activities, in reality they are one and the same thing. Unless you lead two very different lives which begin and end at your front door, it is very difficult to prevent things you learn from your private life experience spilling over into your working life, and vice versa. It is only relatively recently, and because of the increasing use of profiles, that we have realised the benefits of not making false divisions between personal and professional development.

It has been estimated that nurses, midwives and health visitors represent about 80 per cent of the overall workforce in the health service. This force of numbers means that they are the most important resource in making sure the health service achieves its purpose. It also means that if they do not develop as professionals, the service will not develop.

Nursing and midwifery have been striving for professional status for years. It was recognised early on that to achieve this status, nursing and midwifery would need to become research-based activities. Recognition of another characteristic of professional groups – the ability to develop and progress – came more slowly. Such development is achieved not only through the new knowledge gained through research findings, but also through other means such as experiential learning and reflective practice.

Profiles and portfolios

As we identified in Chapter 1, the terms profile and portfolio are often used interchangeably. Nurses and midwives often ask if there is any real difference between a profile and a portfolio, or whether it is just a question of semantics. The producers of profiles and portfolios have added to the problem by selling products that essentially look the same, whilst calling them different names.

A brief look at the literature shows that variation too. Redman (1994) urges us not to make a big song and dance about definitions since 'a portfolio is simply a tangible record of what someone has done'. He does not bother to make a distinction between a profile and a portfolio. Brown (1992) does. She defines the term personal portfolio as:

> a private collection of evidence which demonstrates the continuing acquisition of skills, knowledge, attitudes, understanding and achievement. It is both retrospective and prospective, as well as reflecting the current stage of development of the individual.

She goes on to define a profile as:

> a collection of evidence which is selected from the personal portfolio for a particular purpose and for the attention of a particular audience.

The distinction Brown makes is probably the most useful way of distinguishing between a profile and a portfolio, as it draws on the way people apply the terms in general English usage.

It is difficult to know why and how this differing use of the terms has arisen, and to some extent it does not matter. Having identified that confusion exists, this alerts you to the fact that it is important to find out how someone is using the term so that you are able to share their perceptions before jumping to conclusions.

The way the terms are used often comes from the particular purpose of the profile or portfolio. For example, the term most frequently associated with accreditation of prior experiential learning (APEL) is portfolio preparation.

Most people, if asked what a portfolio is, would probably think of an art portfolio. Indeed Brown (1992) admits that the art portfolio influenced her definition of a portfolio given above. An art portfolio is simply a collection of materials, which aims to demonstrate the owner's artistic development. It can include writing, drawings or sculpture. It can be large or small; it can be thick; it can be thin. Ideally it is not judged in terms of volume, but rather by its relevance and quality. All of this is very close to how a portfolio is used in the APEL context. Significantly enough, the *Oxford English Dictionary* describes a portfolio as follows: 'collection, set, archives, file, record, folder, bundle'.

So, a portfolio of prior learning is simply a record of your past learning and learning achievements. It does not have to be written and it can contain drawings, a computer package, a video or even a sculpture. Indeed, the majority of guidelines for constructing a portfolio do not seek to prescribe what should be included or how it should be presented. So, for example, the English National Board's *Professional Portfolio* clearly states that it has been designed:

> to enable you to keep a record of your personal and professional development, your professional experiences and qualifications . . . The Professional Portfolio is more than a straightforward recording device. It is also a way for you to develop skills of critical reflective practice, to consider experiences in your professional and personal life and to evaluate the contribution those experiences make to your development and to improvements in client care.

Interestingly, the term profile was chosen by those developing the Nursing Times (now Macmillan Open Learning) *Profile Pack*, because they felt the word more accurately portrayed the personal development aspect of profile work. The *Profile Pack* states that profiling is important for two reasons:

- As an individual: understanding and appreciating the significance of what and how you learn involves an ongoing process of reflection which will enhance your self-awareness and build confidence in the value of your life and experience to date.
- As a professional: having an effective and up-to-date

record of your past and current learning and experience will provide you with a powerful means of communication with employers, both present and future.

In this approach, a professional profile is expected to acknowledge the integrity or wholeness of the individual.

Generally speaking there are characteristics which are common to a profile and a portfolio. They both:

- value experience as a source of learning
- encourage reflective practice
- provide a storehouse for information about and evidence of experience, learning and achievements
- encourage personal and professional development.

As stated earlier, we will be using the term 'profile' throughout the book, unless referring to a specific product called a portfolio.

Experiential learning

Whilst experiential learning is often very much part of the assessment of prior learning, its meanings and traditions have a far broader application.

People learn from a wide variety of sources. They learn from relationships with friends, family and colleagues. They learn from social activities such as sport, voluntary work, travel and reading – in fact from almost every activity in which they are involved. However, although people clearly learn from experience, not all experiences lead to learning.

The starting point in discussing what we mean by experiential learning, therefore, is to ask how experience is related to learning. Experiential educators have had many arguments over this question. Nevertheless, nearly all would agree with John Dewey, an American philosopher generally regarded as one of the early key figures in experiential education. Dewey (1933) argues that for experience to become learning it needs to include 'an active and passive element peculiarly combined. On the active hand, experience is trying . . . On the passive it is undergoing.' In other words, for Dewey, learning from experience is making 'backward and forward connections between what we do to things and what we enjoy or suffer from things in consequence'.

In short, in experiential learning the learner is directly involved with the realities being studied. This can be contrasted with learning which is only read, heard, talked or written about, but where the reality of practice is never brought into the learning process.

In more recent times the work of David Kolb (1984) has elucidated the basic principles of experiential learning. Influenced by philosophers such as Dewey, Kolb argues for a relationship between thinking and experience. He views experiential learning as a cycle involving action and reflection, theory and practice. When profiles are used primarily as a *learning* tool, they tend to adopt the framework of Kolb's learning cycle. We shall therefore be returning to explore Kolb's work in greater depth elsewhere.

So far we have said that experiential learning involves not merely theory but practice, not simply observing but doing. This is one of the reasons why it is seen as a particularly effective approach to professional education. As a tool in professional development, experiential learning is certainly not new. Rather, we can see it reflected in the craft guilds and apprenticeship systems that provided so much advanced training from the medieval period through to the industrial revolution. Then, as now, people learnt experientially and informally, whilst at the same time having more formal systems of education provided by monks and clergy in monasteries and churches.

So, in one sense there is nothing startling or revelatory about experiential learning. It is simply that academic and professional education are increasingly recognising its benefits and are therefore seeking to foster approaches to education which build upon and value experiential learning.

Another aspect of experiential learning is the emphasis placed upon links between *affective* and *cognitive* learning. If people really do gain so much quality learning from their life and social situations, they have to acknowledge the importance of their emotions in this process. So, for example, learning is often acquired through highly emotional experiences such as bereavement, falling in love, and divorce. Traditionally affective learning has been disregarded because it appears to be a subjective activity, difficult to assess within formal education. As we shall be emphasising throughout this book, however, affective learning is, in theory, no more difficult to assess than cognitive learning (which is concerned with factual knowledge, comprehension and application).

If personal experiences are genuinely regarded as the substance of learning, then the distinctive boundaries created between academic and professional disciplines become nonsensical and need to be dismantled. It does not make sense to ask learners to experience academically one minute and practically the next, or to think historically in one learning situation and mathematically or medically in the next.

As you can see, experiential learning can therefore refer simply to a technique for developing practice-based education, or it can be associated with a whole philosophy of education which supports the notion of open, learner-centred learning. Many experiential educators see experiential learning as:

> a means by which we cease to fragment our experience and our ways of knowing: for instance, intellectual intuitive, social and behavioural. Through experiential learning cycles and processes, we learn to see underlying patterns and connections, and powerful central themes within larger wholes. Making sense of ourselves in relation to the world is at the centre of experiential learning. (Weil and McGill, 1989)

Reflection

All approaches to experiential learning view action and reflection as the basis for learning. In this sense reflection is taken to mean a collection of activities, which might include simply sitting in a corner mulling over thoughts. It can also be a much more dynamic process which involves writing, discussion and learning from conversations with colleagues and friends.

Reflection is fast becoming recognised as an essential component of professional practice, particularly since the publication of Donald Schon's *The Reflective Practitioner*. In this, Schon (1983) looks at the different ways in which we act and reflect in and on action. Schon challenges the traditional assumption that professional practice is simply the application of a task or a display of relevant knowledge to clearly defined problems. We discuss his ideas more fully in Chapter 5.

Reflection in the context of learning suggests that the reflective practitioner is:

> conducting a conversation with herself. The conversation has a critical edge to it, for the professional is always asking the question: what if . . . ? Being faced with fresh problems to which there is no single answer, and no one right answer, the professional has the responsibility to appraise the situation and formulate an effective strategy. The effective professional has, accordingly, to be continually self-critical. (Barnett, 1992)

In the context of profiling, the concept of reflective practice therefore has two important elements. First and foremost reflection is regarded as an activity which can occur at any time after an experience. Indeed, reflection is viewed as an active process which *turns* the experience into learning. An Australian writer, David Boud, has written extensively on the role of reflection in learning. Boud *et al* (1985) take the view that most people are largely unaware of their internal processes for learning. However, once they become aware and skilled at using them, they are likely to become much more effective practitioners. For Boud, reflection is simply a generic term for the mental activities people carry out in order for learning to occur.

Because of the importance of reflection and action in the development of any approach to the profile process, we look at this in much greater depth in Chapter 5.

Credit Accumulation and Transfer Scheme (CATS)

The Credit Accumulation and Transfer Scheme was established by the Council For National Academic Awards (CNAA) and was originally operated in the polytechnic sector of higher education. Although the principles for the scheme and the credit tariff established by the CNAA have largely been adopted by most universities and colleges of higher education, the way they operate is always at the discretion of each institution.

So, each institution designs and operates its own CAT scheme and, in some cases, a different credit tariff is offered. Because of the separate Scottish system for higher education, Scotland has developed a unique CAT scheme called SCOTCAT. These differences between institutions and countries are often misunderstood; people imagine that there is a national scheme which will make it easy to transfer from one institution to another as a student. Whilst this is so in theory, in practice it is far more complicated than that.

The concept of CATS was first widely introduced to nursing and midwifery education with the launch of the English National Board's framework for continuing education and its Higher Award in 1991. The educational and resource benefits of operating within a CAT scheme became available for the first time to nurses and midwives, because of the creation of a modularised degree programme that allowed prior learning from courses and experience to be credited.

The CAT scheme is based on the principle that appropriate learning should be given academic credit wherever it occurs, provided that it can be assessed. So, a significant aspect of the scheme is the flexibility it allows in the mode of attendance and the locations of study. It also means, in theory, that if you move from one geographical area to another, you can transfer credit from one institution to another. Neither is credit lost if you have a break in your studies.

In reality there are sometimes practical problems encountered by students when they try to get one university to accept credit from another. The problems with implementing a CAT scheme in line with the original philosophy are outlined in the HEQC report (1994). Whilst all universities broadly operate within the higher education system, each university is academically autonomous with very individual missions. This often means that they do not automatically accept the academic decisions of another university, and therefore ease of transfer of credit is prevented. There are also some economic constraints for the students in the transfer of credit, as each university will charge a fee to assess and accredit learning gained elsewhere.

In order to facilitate the transfer of credit, the CNAA devised a credit tariff scheme which is based on the assumption that, to obtain an Honours degree, students must accumulate 360 credit points across three levels of study. In each case the credit points represent the *total* workload required to obtain the award. As well as accumulating credit points, the points need to be obtained at certain levels. Unfortunately each university has its own interpretation of what these levels should be. The only national guidance has been provided by the Council for National Academic Awards (CNAA). (This body was disbanded in 1994 and replaced with the Open University Validation Service.) The CNAA (1989) said that levels 1, 2 and 3 should be based on what was expected of a full-time undergraduate student in their first, second and third years. This brief explanation was not considered to be very helpful by colleges of nursing and midwifery and their associated universities, who were trying to design flexible degree programmes which related to professional practice. The lack of central guidance has led to variations in the way universities interpret the different levels, as James and Redfern (1995) have identified.

Finally, it is important to understand that a distinction is made between **general credit**, which you acquire from previous study, and **specific credit**, which you acquire when you apply your prior credit to a specific programme of studies for a future award. This means that specific credit refers to the use of general credit within your chosen programme of study.

Chapter 6 expands on the terminology of a CAT scheme.

APL and APEL

Accreditation of prior learning (APL) and accreditation of prior experiential learning (APEL) are terms that have become part of nursing and midwifery educational jargon. Understanding of what they mean has now become more widespread, but difficulties still exist. Although the terms are sometimes used synonymously, it is useful to recognise the difference between APL and APEL.

APL, in the nursing and midwifery context, is largely taken to mean formal or informal learning which has not yet been given formal recognition or validation. It can also refer to learning which, whilst already recognised, needs to be reassessed within a different context and for different educational and professional purposes. So, for example, you might have recently finished a short training course or completed an Open University module. On their own, neither of these will give you the qualification you require. Nevertheless, they may stand as proof of your ability to study at a particular level and to show your interest in a particular topic. The learning you acquired from the course may be part of a larger programme you intend to study, and it would be pointless for you to repeat it.

The emphasis in APEL is on experiential learning. This is taken to mean learning which has been acquired informally, unintentionally and from life experience. A large part of the process therefore is in *identifying* and *articulating* this learning in a way that can be assessed by others. A profile can be very useful here – Chapter 6 explains how a profile can be used in the assessing and accrediting process.

If you look back to the early history of APEL in Britain, you will find that it was originally offered as a taught course within an adult education 'access and return to learn programme'. One of the first of these was held at Goldsmiths' College, University of London, in 1984 and is fairly typical of what was on offer at that time. The course was called *Making Experience Count*. It was run over a 20-week period for 3 hours per week. The central purpose of the course was to enable learners to recognise learning which has taken place as a result of different life experiences. 'Each member of the group begins to recognise the richness of the informal learning they have acquired, and through the production of a personal learning portfolio is enabled to convey this to others' (FEU, 1987).

In short, APEL was largely conceived as a self-assessment tool. Through the process of recollection and identification of learning, students were able to recognise personal qualities, knowledge and skills. They were then helped to put this into a form which could be assessed by others. Since that time, this has been taken one step further and the 'A' in APEL now usually refers to accreditation as well as assessment.

Accreditation

A simple definition of accreditation is that it is the *process* of giving formal recognition or validation to skills, knowledge, experience or competence. In short, it is giving public recognition to what you already know and can demonstrate. It might be useful at this point to remind you that whilst assessment and accreditation are closely connected, they are not the same. Although learning cannot be accredited without being assessed, clearly learning can be assessed without being accredited.

Learning outcomes

The increasing use of learning outcomes has been one way in which a variety of professions, professional and accrediting bodies have sought to create a balance between giving recognition to what people can *do* and allowing them to develop their own private record of ongoing personal development. At their simplest, learning outcomes are a clearly worked out description of what people need to demonstrate they have achieved in order to have their learning assessed, usually against a particular qualification or award.

Learning outcomes are also used by course developers to show the intention of the programme. For example, each module will have a set of learning outcomes which need to be achieved. This is helpful when you are going to use evidence from your profile to show which parts of the programme you do not need to repeat. Another approach is to make clear to learners what they are being assessed against, but to do so in a way that does not *prescribe* what should be included and allows them to articulate qualities and knowledge, as well as skills, from their own perspective. So, for example, the *Professional Portfolio* has been designed as an integral part of the ENB framework for continuing professional education for nurses and midwives. The framework is based on ten key characteristics which represent areas of skill, knowledge and expertise that 'all nurses midwives and health visitors must have in order to provide the quality of care required to meet the changing health care needs of the public' (ENB, 1991).

Finally, another approach to learning outcomes is through the development of a learning contract. A learning contract is an agreement made between the learner and the assessor, supervisor or tutor about what the outcomes for the profile should be. The important element here is that the learner is at the centre of the assessment process.

References

Barnett, R. (1992) *Learning to Effect*, SRHE/OU: London

Boud, D., Keogh, R. and Walker, D. (1985) *Reflection: Turning Experience into Learning*, Kogan Page: London

Brown, R. A. (1992) *Portfolio Development and Profiling for Nurses*, Quay Publishing Ltd: Lancaster

CNAA (1989) *The Credit Accumulation and Transfer Scheme: Regulations*, CNAA: London

Dewey, J. (1933) *How We Think*, DC Health and Co: Boston

ENB (1991) *ENB Framework for Continuing Professional Education for Nurses, Midwives and Health Visitors: Guide to Implementation*, ENB Publications: London

ENB (1991) *Professional Portfolio*, ENB Publications: London

ENB (1994) *Creating Lifelong Learners: Partnerships for Care*, ENB Publications: London

FEU (1987) *Aspects of Assessing Experiential Learning: Case Studies*, FEU Publications: London

James, C. and Redfern, L. (1995) 'The description of levels in nursing degrees: an illustration and analysis of the variations', *Journal of Clinical Nursing*, 4, 311–17

HEQC (1994) *Choosing to Change: The Report of the HEQC CAT Development Project*, HEQC Publications: London

Kolb, D. (1984) *Experiential Learning: Experience as a Source of Learning and Development*, Prentice Hall: New Jersey

Macmillan Open Learning (1994) *Profile Pack*, Macmillan Magazines: London

Redman, W. (1994) *Portfolios for Development: A Guide for Trainers and Managers*, Kogan Page: London

Schon, D. (1983) *The Reflective Practitioner*, Basic Books Inc: New York

UKCC (1994) *The Future of Professional Practice and Education: The Council's Standards for Education and Practice Following Registration*, UKCC: London

Weil, S. and McGill, I. (eds) (1989) *Making Sense of Experiential Learning*, SRHE/OU Press: London

Some Common Themes and Questions Shared 3

This chapter will help you to think about what you need to begin developing your profile. We explore the ten most common questions people ask, including:

- Why do I need to compile a profile?
- Should I buy a ready-made profile?
- How do I decide which profile to buy?
- How long will it take to complete?

When you begin developing your profile, it usually feels like uncharted territory. Being asked to reflect upon your life experience feels endless and overwhelming. These are some of the most common comments made:

- 'I am 48. I've been around for a long time. That's a lot of experience to think about. I don't know where to start.'
- 'I haven't done anything significant. I haven't any experiences worth reflecting on.'
- 'It feels frightening. I am worried it is going to throw up feelings I would rather forget.'
- 'I don't know what it is you are looking for.'
- 'It's wonderful. I've not stopped thinking about myself all week.'

- 'I didn't realise I had done so much. I didn't realise I had so much to offer.'
- 'What has been surprising to me is how interesting it is. I've never really thought about what I have done before or how I feel.'
  (Comments made by students attending profile classes, Goldsmiths' College, University of London, 1992)

For some people the process can seem daunting because they have lived and learnt so much; whereas some are lost because they feel they have not lived or learnt at all. They might feel excited by thinking about their experiences, often for the first time; but by opening themselves up in this way, they also fear they could expose themselves to feelings and emotions which they would rather forget, or which will leave them feeling vulnerable. In addition, whilst feeling good about recognising the extent of their own experience and learning, some people feel unsure about what an assessing panel or awarding body is looking for and whether the learning they identify is relevant or at an appropriate standard.

In the next chapter we explore some of these issues and offer practical suggestions as to how you might work effectively through the profile process. Because each profile is unique, each person will approach its construction in different ways. This, in turn, means that each person will have unique issues and questions which they need to address as they begin work. To help you to identify some of these issues, therefore, this chapter explores the ten most common questions asked initially about profiling. Within each of these you will wish to identify a subset of questions and issues of your own. You will find that there are few right or wrong answers. Rather, you will need to think about how you work best and decide which is the right answer for you. The views expressed here are those held by the authors – be prepared to question what is being said, and to contribute a few ideas of your own.

Why do I need to compile a profile?

Throughout this book we stress that profiling provides a flexible approach to professional development, offering people greater choice over what they want to learn and how they want to develop as health care professionals. However, many practitioners argue that profiling actually limits choice, as it is now a compulsory element of professional development. From 1995 all nurses, health visitors and midwives will be required to complete a profile in order to register. It is true that, by making profiling a compulsory component of registration, nurses and midwives have little choice as to whether or not to complete it. However, the profile process itself is far from limiting. Rather, it enhances and broadens your opportunities and maximises your personal and professional potential.

It is important to bear in mind that, as a professional, you are responsible for maintaining the effectiveness of your practice. Ideas about the profession in which you are working change continually. As a professional you need to be aware of these ideas and how they impinge on your everyday practices. Within this context, profiling offers maximum choice about what you want to learn and how you want to develop in the future. Profiling, therefore, provides the most appropriate method for addressing professional development needs.

The best profile is one that *supports* your professional development in a number of ways. In particular, it will enable you to develop the skills to reflect upon and critically assess what you know and can do. Once you are able to articulate the range and depth of your learning, both to yourself and to others, you are in a much stronger position to be able to make decisions about courses you wish to attend and the knowledge you want to develop in the future. So, profiling enables you to identify realistic and relevant future educational goals.

Should I buy a ready-made profile?

There are two main reasons why people buy a ready-made profile. The first is that some profiles have been 'tailor made' for a specific purpose and to match a specific set of prescribed learning outcomes. The second is that buying a profile offers a ready-made structure in a professionally designed format.

However, you should not feel obliged to buy a profile off the shelf. Many people can and do create their own well-organised and professional profile. Indeed, some organisations regard the skills required in the personal design of a profile as an integral part of the learning process, and it is sometimes possible to gain accreditation for this additional effort. Developing a profile from scratch simply takes a little more planning at the outset.

How do I decide which profile to buy?

There are many profiles on the market and it is worthwhile investing time in deciding which one is best for you.

Deciding which profile to buy requires the same approach as for choosing any major product. Begin by clarifying your aims and establishing criteria before deciding which is the most appropriate. This will combine common sense and personal preference. For example, when deciding which car to buy, your decisions will be based upon how much driving you do (comfort, cost of petrol, etc); your garage/car space; the image you want to project; maintenance cost; and personal colour preference. When deciding which profile to buy, the areas you need to consider are purpose, accessibility, content, design and layout, and cost.

Purpose

Whether you are buying a profile off the shelf or building your own, the first step is to clarify who you are seeking to communicate with. If, for example, you are seeking to use your profile to apply for a particular job, you will be communicating with colleagues, usually at a more senior level, working in the same profession. If, by contrast, you wish to submit your profile for academic purposes, you will be communicating with academic staff who might be new to your profession and its language. So, whatever your purpose, when embarking on a profile you need to consider how it will be received and, above all, by whom.

Having said this, most people will be developing a profile for two reasons: firstly, to enhance professional development in the broadest terms; secondly, for a range of purposes which might include applying for jobs, access to academic credit, and/or retaining professional registration.

Whatever your purpose, it is important to remember that the profile is a process which enables you to communicate more effectively with yourself and others. The best profile, therefore, is one which provides you with both a private and public record.

A private record: communicating with yourself

Profiling is a system of discovering and recording information about your personal and professional life. Some of the information you choose to include in the profile, therefore, will be sensitive and you will want it to remain private. Through the private record you might also wish to experiment with developing a writing style, or with new ideas and concepts. In addition, you might wish to decide to share your private record with a few, carefully selected people. A good profile, therefore, enables you to record your thoughts privately – perhaps in a way that will only make sense to yourself.

A public record: communicating with others

The vast majority of what you include in the profile will be public. You need to ensure, therefore, that the information you include is easy to read, accessible and well organised.

You will almost certainly wish to include a section about your past employment, education, training and qualifications, as well as biographical details. This might sound like an enhanced curriculum vitae and, in some respects, this is certainly true. However, your professional profile is not simply a record of what you have done; it is also an important record of your personal skills and abilities. Recording these should help you to identify strengths that you did not know you possessed, together with areas you would like to develop and improve. In short, the profile is expected to demonstrate your 'ongoing' professional development. Some profiles have sections and exercises to assist you with this, including the identification of goals and action plans for the future. Others, by contrast, simply refer to a bibliography of suggested reading.

Accessibility

It is essential that the material in the profile you purchase is accessible and has relevance for you. When buying one, you should consider the following:

- Is it written clearly and in a language I can understand?
- Are any difficult terms or concepts clearly explained?
- Is it versatile? Are each of the sections independent of each other, allowing me to move around easily within the material as a whole?
- Are there any guidelines on how to use the materials?
- Are there activities or materials which enable me to reflect upon and evaluate my past as well as current learning?

Content

The reason most people find difficulty in deciding which profile to buy is that they have no clear idea what they want to use it for – they simply know they have to complete one. Once you know what kind of profile you wish to produce, you will find it easier to choose a profile which is best suited to meeting your needs.

In deciding which profile to buy, however, it is important

that you do not opt for the one which appears to provide the softest option, offering very few challenges. Working through exercises which enable you to understand the depth and range of your knowledge is a crucial part of the process. Constructing a profile is not always easy, and is rarely straightforward. Most people who have completed a profile say it is both demanding and time-consuming. They also say that it is well worth the effort and extremely rewarding:

> I found reflecting on my personal life much harder than I had thought it would be. Some of the skills I have learned go as far back in my childhood to when I worked in an old people's home as a Saturday weekend helper. When I began to reflect it felt like an enormous task. Now, I can see it is a skill I've developed. I find it easier to make connections with my past experiences now. In fact I find it exciting to learn more and more about what makes me tick. I can now see the fruits of my labour. I want to continue developing my portfolio forever! (Hull, 1993)

So, when deciding which profile to buy, ask yourself:

- Will this profile challenge me to think?
- Will it enable me to learn more about myself and to make connections with my past and current learning?
- Will it integrate my personal and professional learning?
- Is the content flexible enough for me to use it for a variety of purposes?

Design and layout

The design and layout are important factors to consider, both in terms of presentation and ease of use.

Binder

A profile binder must be sturdy enough to withstand heavy use as you continually put things into it, take things out and move material around within it. In choosing a binder, therefore, consider the following:

- How strong is it: will it stand up to perpetual use?
- Is it the right size in depth and length?
- Does it present the appropriate image?
- Can you carry it around or will it be too bulky?

Dividers

- Will they withstand perpetual use?
- Are they easy to differentiate? (Remember: your profile will eventually be filled with paper.)

Forms

Some profiles provide forms for you to include in your finished document.

- Are they clear and easy to use?
- Are they appropriate (both in level and content)?
- Can they be photocopied easily?
- Can you obtain more copies if necessary?
- Do they look professional?

Workbooks

Some profiles include workbooks and materials.

- Is the language clear and accessible?
- Is the spine strong, or will it crack with perpetual use?
- Will it be easy to use?

Considering the layout is also important.

- Is it attractive and appealing?
- Does it interest you?
- Will you be able to move around the materials easily and can you open the workbook at any point and begin?

General content

- Is there a glossary of terms to help you understand any jargon?
- Is there a bibliography of further reading?
- Are there activities and materials to stimulate your thinking?
- Will any of the information given help you in constructing the profile?
- Are there materials to help you develop your writing skills?
- Does it include a professional record of your formal learning and qualifications?
- How much room is there to include details of your informal, personal and 'on-the-job' learning?
- Is there information on where to go if you need further help?

Cost

Clearly, cost is an important consideration. As with buying any product, the most expensive profile might not necessarily be the best one. Deciding how much to spend will largely be determined by how much you can afford and which profile best fulfils your criteria. At the time of going to press, most profiles cost between £20 and £25. Any more than this and you need to give very careful consideration to the additional benefits.

What can I put into it?

Most people know and can do far more than they think they can. In particular, they barely recognise the extent to which their informal, experiential learning is used in professional practice. This is largely because learning in our culture is so frequently associated with formal qualifications that uncertificated learning, which may often involve considerable effort and expertise, is disregarded. In addition, people often have only a limited functional notion of what their actual work tasks involve. Once you come to recognise that learning is infinitely transferable, you will quickly find that you have a vast store of knowledge and skills to bring to your profile.

How long will it take to complete?

In constructing a profile, it is important to have a structure to work within. However, understanding the different ways in which you wish to use your profile will help you to set one or a series of deadlines for completion. Work on the profile at your own pace, based upon your needs and deadlines. Your profile should become a valuable record of learning which you will wish to return to continuously throughout your career. Building your profile should not be seen as entering a race, but rather as a time for you to spend thinking about your current and future professional development needs.

Who owns my profile?

Your profile is unique to you and will contain personal as well as public information. You have complete ownership of it. Some organisations have now bought profiles for their staff to complete. Whilst this is in the main a positive step, it is important that you establish, from the outset, your ownership of the profile. This means that you retain the right to withhold some of its content. In some cases it might be necessary to clarify this with an employer in advance. If it becomes clear that an employer has the right to demand access to the profile provided, the answer is simple: record all of your private information in a separate file – one bought and owned by you. The UKCC makes it clear what part of your profile it may request to see.

How do I know that the learning I am demonstrating is at the appropriate level?

Clearly not all of what you have learnt is necessarily appropriate for inclusion in your profile. We can all identify learning which, whilst useful in one context, is not useful in another. Before you begin, therefore, you need to make sure that you have a fundamental understanding of the criteria against which your profile is being assessed. To enable this, the professional or academic body which is assessing your profile needs to provide you with clear guidelines and criteria as to what is being expected of you. You can only be sure that what you are demonstrating is of the appropriate standard and quality, if you have a clear idea what the standard and quality should be. Most organisations should be able to provide you with a set of guidelines and criteria upon request.

How much information should I include?

It is natural for people to want to include *everything* they know about a topic in their profile, but this is not practical, feasible or sound educational practice. In most academic and professional examinations the questions are narrowly focused. So, for example, when sitting an A-level English Literature examination, students are not asked to repeat everything they have learnt about the nineteenth-century novel. Rather, they are required to answer 3–4 narrowly focused but carefully constructed questions. The same approach is adopted in profiling. The points to remember are:

- It is your learning and not your experience which is being assessed
- The learning you are demonstrating should be sharply focused against the assessment criteria.
- You are aiming to convince your reader that you can meet the assessment criteria – you are not trying to tell everything you know.

The best profiles, therefore, are not always the most bulky. They are the ones which are *concise* and *direct*. What is essential, however, is that the evidence you provide is authentic – it must be your own work and have meaning for you. This means that you must 'speak with your own voice', using your own phrases and a personal approach to the task.

This might at first appear daunting, but, in reality, once you have developed your writing skills and can write with confidence you will find that your own style is far more effective.

What should I do if I haven't written for a long time?

Profiling is not simply about past and future learning: it also provides an excellent opportunity to develop skills and knowledge. Profiling requires you to use a range of different writing skills. These might be grouped as **formal** and **informal**. Formal writing includes essays, reports, letters requesting references, completion of goal and action plans, and development of learning contracts. Informal writing includes keeping a diary or journal, writing to a colleague or friend, and summaries of ideas, thoughts and feelings.

As you begin to develop your profile, you may need to develop a range of writing skills which are new to you. There are two ways in which you can improve your formal writing skills. Firstly, you can buy one of the many books on study skills currently available on the market. This should give practical advice and ideas, especially about writing essays and reports. In the bibliography there will also be some suggested reading. Secondly, you might prefer to enrol for a taught course and share what you are learning with others. Most institutes of adult education and further education colleges provide short study skills courses. Many of these are offered in the evening and a fee is charged. Attending a course is useful because it offers the opportunity to experiment with different forms of writing, to look at other people's approach and to get independent constructive criticism.

Writing is all about presenting your thoughts, feelings and ideas in a way which can be read and understood by others. If this is to be effective, you need to learn how to write using your own words and phrases, and your own voice. This is why informal writing is so important. The process of *reflecting through writing* will help in the process of reflecting on practice. Committing your thoughts on paper is in itself reflective and, as you develop your skills of reflection, so you develop your ability to write with meaning and clarity. Playing around with words, feeling comfortable with what and how you write, is integral to owning and taking responsibility for your development and learning:

> She must learn again to speak
> starting with I
> starting with We
> starting as the infant does
> with her own true hunger
> and pleasure
> and rage.
> (Marge Piercy, in Belenky *et al* (1986)

Where can I go for help?

Usually, when studying, you are presented with a curriculum. With profiling, *you* are the curriculum and most of the knowledge, skills and qualities required come from yourself. Finding opportunities to discuss your progress with others has many benefits. It enables you to:

- recognise your similarities and differences with others
- articulate your experience
- receive feedback and positive criticism from others
- explore ways of constructing your profile
- develop your presentation skills
- have a regular focus for developing your profile.

There are many people with whom it would be useful to meet in this way. For example, you might wish to share the development of your professional record with a senior colleague. By contrast, if you are exploring a range of aspects of your professional role, you might want to talk with colleagues at a similar level. Some people find it useful to talk with colleagues they work with on a day-to-day basis. Others find it more useful to find a colleague working at some distance, perhaps in a different environment. When you are exploring personal and/or sensitive issues, you need to find people you trust and who will be sympathetic. Most people choose to use family or friends. However, some find it easier to talk with people who are less involved in their lives, but can be trusted to be confidential.

Increasingly, many colleges provide short courses in profiling. Often these courses are attended by people from a wide variety of professional and non-professional backgrounds. Joining a course has the added bonus of a group tutor or facilitator, who should encourage you to keep working. Contact your local library for information on courses that are available in your area.

References

Belenky, M., Clinchy, B., Goldberger, N. and Taroule, J. (1986) *Women's Ways of Knowing: The Development of Self, Voice and Mind*, Basic Books Inc: New York

Hull, C. (1993) 'Making Sense of Profiling', in N. Graves (ed) *Learner Managed Learning: Practice, Theory and Policy*, Higher Education for Capability: Leeds

Getting Started: Creating Your Personal Profile 4

In this chapter you will find practical advice on how to develop a framework for completing your profile. There is information on cross-referencing, layout and presentation. Because writing is an essential part of the process, you will find information on how to develop your writing skills. We also include suggestions on how to write clear statements of competence to support examples of what you can do, together with advice on how to present your work in a way which can be easily understood and assessed by others.

This chapter has been designed to enable you to work at your own pace. You can move backwards and forwards within it, according to which aspect of your profile you are working on. Although we have included activities and practical materials, you will find additional resources in the Annotated Bibliography.

Constructing a coherent profile requires you to be able to carry out a number of different tasks simultaneously. At any one time you might be reflecting upon your past experience; writing letters to potential referees; developing your writing skills; thinking about your future educational needs; and keeping a private record of your thoughts and feelings. Although this might seem daunting, it is actually fairly simple. This is because each task often dovetails and is dependent upon another. As each section is completed it will be cross-referenced with the rest of the text. Each piece of writing, therefore, needs to be free-standing, whilst at the same time continually integrated with the rest of the material you are producing.

The profile process therefore involves a series of interlocking and yet separate stages which include taking stock; developing a structure; reflecting on past learning; identifying significant learning; proving what you know and can do; and constructing your profile. We will now be exploring each of these in depth. Although activities have been incorporated into the text, additional resources can be found in the Annotated Bibliography. These will give you more ideas for how you can work through each stage.

You do not have to work through each of these stages consecutively. Rather, you should use the sections which best suit your needs as you are working on your profile.

Taking stock

> Tell me and I forget
> Teach me and I remember
> Show me and I understand
> (Chinese proverb)

People learn through an active engagement in a four-stage process, which includes personal experience; reflection; making connections between what they are learning and what they know; and experimentation or testing. There are a great many other factors, however, which affect how people learn. These include cultural roots and identity, environmental factors, motivation, previous experiences of learning, emotional and anxiety factors. So, for example, some people may have had bad schooling experiences. They might have been made to feel stupid at not being able to accomplish specific tasks. They might have felt bored and disinterested with school. Their culture and personal identity may have gone unrecognised, and they may have felt confused or isolated by reading texts which had no direct relevance to their own experiences. For some people then, their experiences of learning have left them with negative feelings about their own capabilities and learning generally. Such people may continue to think that they are stupid, rather than acknowledge the failure of the education system in assisting them to learn. They may believe their early boredom at school signified that they were simply not good at learning, rather than being the fault of an education system that failed to motivate and challenge.

Beginning a profile allows you to consider how you prefer to learn, to think about what stops you learning and how this can be overcome. You will be simultaneously reflecting upon your past experience (of school), working out how you learn best (when the learning is made relevant and recognises your identity), and beginning to create a framework from which to develop your profile.

Reflecting on past experiences

Reflecting on past experiences can clearly be an enormous task. In the Annotated Bibliography you will find references to materials which will help you with this process, but it is important to remember that you can create your own ways of doing this.

Looking through old photographs is often a useful starting point. Photographs can be the key to unlocking many memories. They may remind you of friends you have long forgotten and places you once visited. They can also reflect your physical changes, moods and the different roles you have undertaken throughout your life. Alternatively, you may find it useful to create a lifeline which charts different aspects of your life such as chronological dates, places you have visited, people you have known, colours and smells you like and dislike, and happy and sad times. The lifeline activity is described in more depth on page 56. If you prefer making things, you may find that you are better able to picture your experiences through painting or sculpture.

Whichever way you approach it, as you begin to put

together the jigsaw puzzle of your life, you will find that you remember events you have long forgotten – events which you particularly enjoyed and had meaning for you. This is useful in assessing your learning, as well as in clarifying your aspirations for the profile. Very often people presume that what they formally achieved at school is what they are naturally good at and interested in. But this is not always the case.

CASE STUDY: Marian

Marian joined the profile course because she wanted to be a nursery nurse. As she did not have the correct qualifications, she wanted to use the profile course as an alternative access route. Before she started she said that she wanted to do this because she had been bringing up three children for the last 12 years and felt that she had a lot of experience which would equip her for becoming an effective nursery nurse.

As she began to take stock of her life, there could be no doubt that she did, in fact, have a wealth of relevant experience for nursery nursing. At the same time, however, she began to reflect upon other experiences and interests which she had either forgotten or had not pursued.

This led her to realise that, having brought up children for the last 12 years, the last thing she really wanted to do was return to work to nurse young children. Rather, what she wanted to do was train to become a florist. This was something she had thought about many years previously, but, having raised her children, she had pushed it out of her mind. In fact, she found that she didn't need to complete her profile in order to become a trainee florist. Nevertheless, she found the process had developed her confidence enormously and went on to complete it.

Since then Marian has been offered a job as a trainee florist and has now qualified.

In this case study, Marian's reasons for developing a profile changed as she began to assess her true interests and aspirations. Although she did not need to do so, Marian chose to complete her profile because it had given her confidence. The framework she created, therefore, was very different to the one she originally envisaged, which was organised around meeting the specific criteria for nursery nursing. Her profile acquired a much more personal approach.

At this early stage in the development of your profile, you need to reflect on experiences that you think are important because you:

- think you have learnt a lot
- are pleased with what you feel you have achieved
- have received recognition
- have put in considerable time and effort
- have found the experience either positive or enjoyable
- have found the experience peculiarly negative, or disturbing in some way.

Some of the aspects of your life you might find useful to explore are:

Work   This means thinking about the paid and unpaid jobs you have done

Voluntary activities   This can include involvement in political activities, work with community groups, charity work, public service or fundraising.

Educational activities   Most people can identify an in-service training course they have attended. However, you also learn from evening classes you have taken, television programmes you have watched, Open University courses you have studied but did not finish, and lectures and seminars you have attended.

Travelling   This includes travelling for both work and pleasure.

Hobbies   These include leisure activities such as gardening or going to the theatre, as well as more organised hobbies such as sports or playing a musical instrument.

Relationships Consider relationships which have had meaning for you.

Other Other aspects of your life worth exploring might include caring for others, books you have read, and projects you have carried out. The list is endless!

As with Marian (in the case study above) your approach to, and goals for, the profile may change during the course of its development. Through reflecting upon your learning, you will come to realise that you are good at many activities, and that you have been in the business of learning for a long time and have learnt a great deal. You will be able to identify many skills and pieces of knowledge that will enable you to access a range of job or educational possibilities.

At some point at this early stage, you need to remind yourself of your real reasons for developing the profile. Here are the most commonly cited reasons:

- to clarify my career and/or educational goals
- to gain access to job opportunities
- to gain access to educational opportunities
- to get credit against college courses.

You might wish to include more than one of these reasons in your personal list for developing your profile.

A focus on personal and professional development

Profiling is an excellent opportunity for you to take stock of your life and career in the context of your future educational- and work-related goals. Some people may already have given a great deal of thought to their future career. The vast majority, however, whilst wishing to develop their career, have not spent time focusing on the direction they would like to take.

It is always worth investing time in carefully reviewing your situation and ensuring that the choices are genuine, realistic and achievable. So, for example, Sarah decided that she wanted to do a profile because:

> I have been bringing up children for five years. I have learnt a lot about children and I think I would make a good pre-school playgroup leader. A profile would offer me a chance to get on a course as I don't have the right qualifications.

After reviewing her life and experience, however, she changed her mind:

> On reflection, I have been bringing up children for five years. I now feel it is my time and would like to do something different. Although I do enjoy working with youngsters, I think what I have been interested in all my life, and have never had the chance to explore, is English literature. Perhaps I might be an English teacher one day. (Hull, 1993)

Because most people spend their lives juggling the demands of work and home, spending time thinking about their own needs is a luxury they feel they can ill afford. But, taking time to think about who and what you are is important, for both your personal and professional development. It allows you to think about how fulfilled you are at work and whether you wish to move into different areas. Nowadays it is perfectly possible to develop a second career well into your 40s and 50s. As professions change, it is also possible to move into different jobs within the same profession.

Reflection also enables you to make changes in your personal life. You might find that you are unhappy with the balance between home and work. You might be very happy and fulfilled at work but wish you could find a hobby or social life outside of it. At this stage, therefore, you are looking at how the profile process can lead to greater personal and professional satisfaction.

There are many activities which have been designed to help you take stock of your learning and identify your reasons for completing the profile. The following two activities will help you in reviewing your life to date.

ACTIVITY: the lifeline

This will enable you to identify significant events or interests you might wish to explore in the future. Your lifeline will be personal to you and should be kept within the private record section of your profile. It is an activity that can take as long as you feel is appropriate – try not to rush it.

On a piece of paper, represent your life. Do this in a way that has most meaning for you. You might choose to note down important stages and landmarks in your life. You can draw shapes and use colours which reflect important aspects of your life, including places, objects, people and ideas that have influenced you. Some people like to do intricate, colourful drawings, whilst others prefer to draw simple lines or to write. Some use large sheets of coloured paper, whilst others prefer standard A4 white. The important thing is to ensure that it is your personal lifeline which is represented.

Once this has been completed, spend time looking and thinking carefully about what you have produced. Try and identify what is particularly significant to you. It might be, for example, that you have included a particular event which you had long forgotten, but was clearly significant. You might be surprised by what you have left out or how you have represented your life.

This activity is designed to help you to take stock of your experience. It should act as a valuable trigger to memories and past experience, but it should also enable you to recognise how you have grown and developed to date.

The lifeline is something which many people return to continually as they work through their profile. Some update them and reproduce a different lifeline as they continue to develop and learn more about themselves. It is important that each time you have finished working on your lifeline, you think about it and consider what you have gained from doing it.

When making decisions about your future career, you also need to think about the personal values and interests you must satisfy in order to be fulfilled and happy in what you choose to do. Your values affect how you communicate with others and they will have a strong influence on the personal and professional decisions you make. So, you need to take into account what is really important to you when you are making decisions about your career or lifestyle. Of course, values can, and do, change according to age, social and work situation, and interests. Being aware of these changes will enable you to continually reassess what direction you wish your life to take.

ACTIVITY: professional values

Below is a list of 17 values which relate to professional practice. Some will be more important to you than others. Rank the values in order of importance for you (1 being most important, 16 being least important). You may find that you change your mind continually as you progress.

_____ *Promotion* Having the opportunity to excel in your job and to be promoted

_____ *Money* Earning a decent salary; having the opportunity to earn money through overtime and outside of work if necessary.

_____ *Working conditions* Your day-to-day working environment.

_____ *Hours* Working hours to suit your needs and interests (this might include weekends, full-time, part-time, etc).

_____ *Helping clients* Enabling others to improve the quality of their lives.

_____ *Relationships* Working as a team; working well with others; developing friendships with colleagues.

_____ *Recognition* Having your skills and knowledge recognised and appreciated; being taken seriously and given credit for a job well done.

_____ *Learning* Enjoying learning new skills and knowledge, both outside and within the context of work.

_____ *Security* Ensuring you have a job which does not carry the threat of redundancy.

_____ *Time* Having the time to pursue interests outside of work.

_____ *Stress-free work* Work which is free of pressure, anxiety and deadlines.

_____ *Diversity* A job which offers the chance to do different kinds of work, and develop new skills and work in different ways.

_____ *Freedom* Having the freedom to make decisions; to have maximum control over your day-to-day work.

_____ *Admiration* Carrying out work which others will admire you for.

_____ *Manager* Managing and organising the work of others; developing policies and implementing procedures.

_____ *Practitioner* Practising your profession; working with clients, patients, and others.

_____ *Other* Values which are important to you.

Now spend some time looking through the list. What are the factors which may affect the way you approach any future career changes or your professional development? You might find it useful to consider how much your current job fulfils your values and what changes you would like to make in the future.

In this activity you have been looking at values which relate to work and are tangible. However, most values, attitudes and beliefs are not so easy to define because they are more abstract. To gain a comprehensive picture of yourself, therefore, you need to ask questions which help you to understand far more about yourself as a learner and the values you hold. Developing a personal construct grid is one activity which will help you to focus on how you perceive and make judgements about other people. Through this you will be able to focus in more depth on your personal and professional values, attitudes and beliefs.

Profiling encourages you to take stock of yourself in the broadest possible terms. Through construct grids, for example, you will be able to think critically about values and attitudes which inform and underpin your professional practice. In this way, you will not just simply identify your skills and knowledge, you will also come to understand yourself as a learner. This is an essential part of the profiling process. It is our belief that, in order to become an autonomous reflective practitioner, you need to become an autonomous, reflective learner. This means having the ability to reflect upon what you are learning and to make sense of its relevance for you.

Preparation

During this early (planning) stage, there are several factors which you need to consider before beginning work. These are largely to do with time management and creating a learning environment.

Time management

Once you have begun to develop an action plan for completing your profile, you will need to make decisions as to how much time it will take to complete.

If you are using your profile to gain access to a job or course, you will be restricted by an entry or closing date. Knowing that you have to complete your work within a certain time will help you in beginning to plan what can be achieved on a weekly or monthly basis. If you are not restricted by time, you might choose to impose your own deadlines for completion. Of course, you might prefer to work outside a time framework and in a different way. Whatever approach you take needs to be flexible and, most of all, realistic, if it is to be effective. In planning, it is useful to think about the following:

Working life Whether you are working full- or part-time, you need to recognise the amount of time which your working life consumes. This cannot be calculated by the amount of hours spent at work – some people need time to wind up or wind down as they go to and return from work.

Family commitments It is difficult to assess how much time is taken up with the responsibilities of family life. You can work out how much time you spend on chores such as cooking, shopping or cleaning, but finding time to talk with and enjoy the company of close family and friends is much more difficult. Many people find it difficult to create the right balance. You need to allow yourself time to get this right.

Social life Some people may be completing their profile within an agreed time limit. Others, by contrast, will have no fixed limit. Whatever your circumstances, you will need to decide how much time you can realistically give on a weekly basis. Most people are unrealistic when planning deadlines. Because they wish to complete the work as quickly as possible, for example, they drive themselves too hard. So, when they are not able to keep to the deadlines, they feel frustrated and give up.

Allow yourself time to:

- **work**: paid and unpaid
- **rest**: sleep and relaxation
- **play**: with friends and family
- **study**: to complete your profile.

At face value you might feel there is no time left to study, but in reality there is always more time than you think.

ACTIVITY: time management

Make a list of 15 activities which you have carried out over the past month. In this list include daily tasks such as shopping, cleaning and going to the bank, as well as leisure activities such as talking with friends on the telephone, going for a walk or painting a picture. When you have done this, prioritise your activities. Reflect on how much time you have spent on each. Is there a balance between work, rest and play? Can you cut down on the time spent on any of these activities? Can any of them be eliminated?

One way to keep a continuous eye on the time you take to study is to use a 24-hour clock grid:

	12 1 2 3 4 5 6 7 8 9 10 11 12 1 2 3 4 5 6 7 8 9 10 11
Mon	
Tues	
Wed	
Thurs	
Fri	
Sat	
Sun	

Use the grid to help you keep a record of how you spend your time. On a weekly basis, work out how much time you have spent studying. Think about when and where that study has taken place. Has it been concentrated in one- or two-hourly bursts, or have you attempted to fit in your study at 15-minute intervals? Are you spending more than two hours studying at any one time? Most of all, continually reflect on the effectiveness of your study time. Try and work out new ways of working which are best suited to you and your personal situation. This might mean juggling your existing patterns of waking and sleeping.

Once you have decided how much time you will spend developing your profile, you then need to decide *when* to study. Some people prefer to get up early each morning, others prefer to work into the night or at weekends, while many prefer to keep the weekends free to play and relax. Whatever you decide upon, try and stick to at least one fixed point on a weekly basis. This will give you a realistic structure from which to develop.

Environment

Creating your own space to read, write and learn is important. You might be lucky enough to have a study of your own, but, if not, you can create a personal space in your bedroom, dining or spare room. Creating a workspace means thinking about what makes you feel relaxed when you want to learn. This might simply mean putting personal photographs or artifacts on your desk or table. You might prefer a cluttered desk or a table with nothing on it at all. There are no right or wrong answers. What is important is that you feel you are working in your own space, free from interruptions and surrounded by things you need to enable you to study. If it helps, put a *do not disturb* notice on the door during your study period.

Developing a structure

Most people have an idea of the deadline for completing their profile. This might be linked to the date for:

- re-registration
- submitting an application to join a course
- submitting a job application.

Once you know the date for submitting your profile, you will be able to develop a realistic framework for work. You need to work out what needs to be done and how this can be achieved – referred to as the development of a critical pathway. Remember, when doing this, you need to allow time for holiday, social and unforeseen events. Each profiler will have a different way of tackling the task. Your plan might look something like this:

Submission of profile for entry to degree course at Maryfield College: 1 October

20 September
- Submit profile: 1 week early!

15 September
- Final typing
- Revise profile
- Check references, language and accuracy
- Check all testimonials are in

10 September
- Share final draft with partner/colleague or academic friend

Summer holidays

30 August
- Complete profile

---

2 July
- Plan construction of the profile: sequence of work/what should be included

30 June
- Sharpen up writing skills
- Review progress
- Complete goal and action plan to identify strengths and areas of weakness
- Include strengths in profile
- Include reasons why courses applied for will enable weaknesses to be addressed

20 June
- Begin writing required competencies, skills

10 June
- Identification of specific knowledge and skills relating to competencies and knowledge required by college

9 June
- Ensure in receipt of all documentation, including list of competencies, or guidelines and regulations from the college
- Feedback from academic friend on writing skills
- Practise writing in reflective journal

20 May
- Submit new piece of writing for critical review by academic friend

18 April
- Begin writing for references and testimonials

10 April
- Complete goal and action plan to identify and work on strengths and weaknesses in relation to competencies required by the college

18 March
- Begin identifying personal knowledge, skills and experience in relation to competencies and knowledge required by college

Easter holidays

3 March
- Begin understanding competencies and knowledge required by college

15 March
- Work on developing writing skills
- Complete one written piece of work to personal satisfaction

28 February
- Complete activities relating to identification of skills, knowledge and experience

5 February
- Assess effectiveness of personal writing
- Identify where you can go for extra help

12 January
- Begin developing confidence in writing skills
- Write three different pieces of work in reflective diary

10 January
- Spend time reflecting and taking stock of your past experiences, knowledge and skills
- Think about what you have learnt from your experience

5 January
- Begin goal and action plan to identify why you are applying for this course
- What do you need to achieve before completing your profile?

If you have not studied for a long time you might feel you need to brush up or develop your writing skills. Your reflective diary should help you to practise different writing styles and to discover how you prefer to write. There are also many study skills books available to help you (see Annotated Bibliography for more information). However, it is important to remember that the profile is about you and your learning – any writing and reflective skills used should be yours and not copied from a book.

Reflecting on past learning

By now you should have identified why you want to complete a profile and which one will be used, planned your time, created your own personal space, and begun to identify what skills you will need to work on. You should now be able to move into the next stage of work, which we have called 'reflecting on past learning'.

Until now you have been taking stock of your past experiences whilst, at the same time, looking to your future personal and professional goals. The benefits of this are enormous and should not be underestimated. For many it is the first time they have been encouraged to think about themselves in this way. As one woman said, 'My secret dream is that one day I shall go to college. I told my husband this once and he laughed. He thinks college is for brainboxes. This is the first time I have begun to think it might become more than a dream' (Hull, 1993).

At this stage, you will begin to identify the knowledge and skills you have gained from these experiences. Remember, it is not the experience itself which is important, but the learning you have gained from it. Clearly, much of what you have learnt from your experiences has been acquired unconsciously or unintentionally. So, until you spend time carefully thinking and reflecting upon a specific experience, you may well be unaware of how much you have learnt.

You might have already begun to identify some experiences which appear to have been significant for you in some way. For example, as we noted earlier, many people

Figure 4.1 Documenting experience

Date	Place	Experience	Significant learning
Example 1.6.74	St John's Nursery Sidcup	Nursery nurse placement	Working in a team Working on own initiative First aid course Developing writing skills

Figure 4.2 The development process

Experience	Key factors	What I learnt	Using what I have learnt
Example Working as a nursery nurse, St John's Nursery	Looking after children Introducing children to new ideas and ways of playing together Working as a team with other workers Time management Management of self	How to work on my own initiative Some basic skills in facilitating learning Much better at working in a team Better at dealing with crises	Bringing up my own children As a student, able to cope with working under pressure In seminars, much better at learning from and with others Organising my time Listening to others

find that their childhood experiences of school can lead to either a negative or positive attitude towards future learning opportunities. It is these 'significant experiences' to which you need to turn your attention. It is often useful to 'brainstorm' the experience to find out how it has significance for your profile. Figures 4.1 and 4.2 will provide a useful guide in helping you to achieve this.

Identifying significant learning

You will then move on to discover the nature of the learning which has taken place. In thinking about the experience, you want to identify the:

- **knowledge**: what you know
- **skills**: what you can do
- **qualities**: which underpin your knowledge and actions.

At this stage you are doing this primarily in order to assess yourself and to determine your objectives for completing the profile. In the Annotated Bibliography you will find some resources to help you with this process. However, it is not always easy to analyse experiences in this way. Here are three of the most common difficulties expressed.

How do I recognise that learning has taken place?

Much of what you learn occurs unconsciously, unintentionally and outside of formal education and training. So, even when you think about it, it is not always clear what you have learnt from an experience. Until you begin to reflect critically upon your experiences, you will remain unaware of the extent of your learning. As we have said repeatedly, reflection is therefore a crucial element in the learning process and the more you practise the better you become at it. By far the most effective way of reflecting is through journal and diary writing. We discuss this in more detail in Chapter 5.

How can I determine the level of my learning?

Clearly the depth and breadth of your learning will vary depending upon the nature of the experience and the extent to which you have been able to conceptualise and reflect. Learning is largely referred to in levels when it is applied to education and training programmes. The onus is upon the particular awarding body or organisation to clarify the criteria for each level or standard and the skills, knowledge and qualities which are included. When you have a clear idea of this, you can then begin to identify which level your learning can be matched up against. We discuss levels of learning in more depth on page 74.

I do not know how to articulate my learning

One of the most common remarks made by those constructing a portfolio is 'I know what I know but I simply cannot write it.' You might have had a similar experience when trying to draw a picture or play a musical instrument: your hands will not do what your brain is telling them. In reality, this usually means you need to understand more about the nature of the activity and to develop your skills. The key in representational drawing, for example, lies in looking at what is in front of you. Without this skill you will find that when you try to draw a tree, rather than representing what you see, you will create your *idea* of a tree. This is a very different form of art! One of the key skills in constructing a profile is the ability to communicate in different ways and at different levels. Remember, your profile is essentially an act of communication between yourself and another person or persons.

Making connections and testing learning

Through profiling you are being encouraged to reflect upon your experiences from new and different perspectives. This, in turn, can lead you to recognise learning which you might otherwise have overlooked. However, the learning you identify is not always easy to categorise or fit into a logical list of skills and competencies. This is particularly true when the profile process challenges you beyond what you actually did, to think about the learning you needed in order to do it. If, for example, you can say that you have effectively managed a speech therapy clinic at your local health centre, you are also being asked to think about what skills or knowledge you need in order to manage a speech therapy clinic. You might identify some of the following:

- **knowledge**: of speech therapy
- **understanding**: of the needs of your clients
- **ability**: to organise your time in order to meet with each client
- **ability**: to write reports, fill in forms and communicate with other colleagues.

The list is endless – managing a speech therapy clinic is clearly a complicated task. When you are producing your profile, therefore, you need to be clear as to which skills, qualities and knowledge you are seeking to identify. As APEL increasingly becomes part of professional development and national credit systems, more and more organisations should be able to describe clearly the kinds of knowledge, skills and qualities which are required in a profile. The criteria can refer to the outcomes of learning or to the process of learning itself.

As you begin to identify what you have learnt from your experience, you will begin to make connections between this new learning and your existing theories, ideas and knowledge. Learning then becomes more than a narrow, personal view or feeling. Rather, you are connecting it within a much broader framework of knowledge. In academic terms you are 'conceptualising'. This does not mean that your learning no longer has personal meaning. Indeed, it often assumes greater significance, as it is integrated not only with your existing knowledge but also with your personal values, attitudes and beliefs. As with each stage of the profile process, it can also lead to new learning. Let us look at how this works in practice.

CASE STUDY: John

In recalling his childhood, John, a nurse, wrote about being brought up by his grandmother. He described his grandmother as 'full of life' – an intelligent, articulate woman who had championed many causes and undertaken numerous voluntary activities. He said that she was 'more than a mother to me' and that from her he had learnt to respect and give love to others. At this stage his memories were happy and positive. However, in later life his grandmother suffered from a form of senile dementia. John said that she 'no longer appeared to be the woman he had known', but he continued to respect and love her, just as she had taught him. At times they still shared 'special moments' of closeness. There were also times when he could sense her real pain and anxiety as her sharp mind was made aware of her situation. At this stage his memories were much sadder and less positive. What John found particularly disturbing was watching how the professional staff caring for her no longer treated his grandmother with respect. When she was there they would talk about her, but not to her. Decisions were made on her behalf with no explanation. They would speak to her in tones which were patronising. John saw a rapid decline in his grandmother's spirits. When she died he said that she had simply 'lost the will to live'.

Reflecting on this experience, John felt angry about the way his grandmother had been treated. As a nurse he began to connect this experience with his knowledge and experience in caring for the elderly. He started to read papers and articles on care in the community. He came to recognise that not all those caring for the elderly have shared his experience and are sensitive to the needs of others. He came to realise that his professional practice had been informed largely by the values, attitudes and beliefs he had acquired through experiencing his grandmother's illness and subsequent death. At this stage John was making connections between his personal experience and a wider framework of knowledge by:

- reflecting upon his experience
- attending to his feelings about that experience
- identifying what he had learnt from the experience
- relating what he had learnt to theories, knowledge and ideas
- talking his ideas and theories through with others, including colleagues and friends
- reading papers and articles to gain a broader perspective on his experience.

As demonstrated in this case study, profiling is very much concerned with the current learning which you acquire:

- through reflecting upon your past experiences
- as you develop the new skills needed in order to construct your profile, such as communication skills and techniques in reflection and self-assessment
- as you develop new theories and ideas from reading beyond your personal experience.

However, your knowledge and skills are not wholly learnt until you have tested them out in some way.

> One must learn by doing the thing
> For though you think you know it
> You have no certainty until you try.
> (Sophocles)

For your learning to 'be truly learnt' it must be borne out in practice. You can do this in a variety of ways. At times people choose to test learning in 'real life' situations. For others this raises ethical issues and they might choose instead to conduct experiments which simulate the conditions. Very often you will choose a combination of both. You have many options including:

- writing an essay or report
- conducting an experiment (work-based or other)
- drawing a picture
- role playing.

The option you select will depend upon:

- your preferred methods of learning
- the nature of the learning you are reinforcing
- ethical issues
- whether you are learning independently or have a group of peers with whom you can act out your ideas and theories
- the criteria against which your learning is to be assessed.

In the FHE Curriculum Development Project, Judith Hinman and Maggie Hollingsworth use the example shown in Figure 4.3 to demonstrate how development through the profile process can be related to the learning cycle we have just been discussing (FEU, 1987).

Figure 4.3 Example showing how development through the profile process can be related to the learning cycle

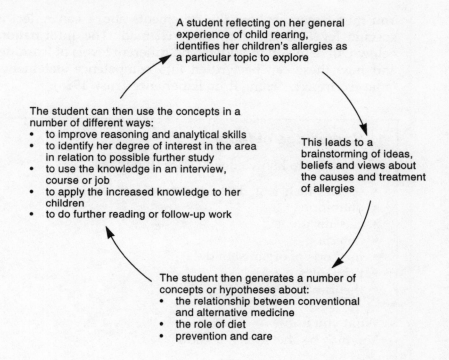

A student reflecting on her general experience of child rearing, identifies her children's allergies as a particular topic to explore

This leads to a brainstorming of ideas, beliefs and views about the causes and treatment of allergies

The student then generates a number of concepts or hypotheses about:
- the relationship between conventional and alternative medicine
- the role of diet
- prevention and care

The student can then use the concepts in a number of different ways:
- to improve reasoning and analytical skills
- to identify her degree of interest in the area in relation to possible further study
- to use the knowledge in an interview, course or job
- to apply the increased knowledge to her children
- to do further reading or follow-up work

Proving what you know and can do

It is important that you express your learning in a way which indicates your learning competence. You can do this by writing clear statements supported by examples of what you can do. An example of a statement of this kind could be:

1 I can extract relevant information from various types of sources, such as books, reports, the media, graphs, and accounts.
2 I can decide the best way to present information for a variety of uses or purposes.
3 I can present information effectively in the form of oral and written reports, graphs and statistical tables.

Producing competence statements: levels of learning

You might wonder how the statements above can reflect a specific level of learning being claimed. The information below will help you to understand different levels of learning and how these can be written into competence statements (adapted from Learning from Experience Trust, 1988).

---

1. Knowledge of facts

This relates to knowledge of such things as:

- specific facts (e.g. dates, events, places, etc.)
- definitions
- classifications
- criteria
- methods of organising data
- principles
- theories.

What you know
You may be able to say, 'I know:

- the countries in the EC
- the principles of management
- the definition of a contract
- how to solve problems.'

What you can do
What can you do with this knowledge? At the most basic level, you are able to tell others what you know, so you are able to say, 'I can:

- list/name/specify/enumerate the countries in the EC
- recount/repeat the principles of management
- define a contract
- state the techniques of problem solving.'

---

2. Interpretation of factual knowledge

This is rather higher level of learning, because now you can interpret the facts you know both for your own benefit and that of others. It addresses the question, 'Do I understand?'

What you understand
You might answer, 'I understand:

- the EC
- the principles of management
- the definition of a contract
- how to solve problems.'

What you can do
So you are able to say, 'I can:

- describe the countries of the EC
- restate/explain the principles of management
- explain the definition of a contract
- explain the techniques of problem solving.'

3. Application of knowledge

You might be able to go further and apply what you know to concrete situations.

What you understand
'I understand:

- the EC
- the principles of management
- the definition of a contract
- how to solve a problem.'

What you can do
'I can:

- draw a map of the countries of the EC
- locate the EC countries on a map of the world

- apply the principles of management to my department
- draw up a contract
- give examples of a contract
- solve different types of problems.'

4. Analysis of knowledge

At a higher level, you may be able to analyse the knowledge you have (i.e. break it up into its constituent elements) in a variety of ways and for a variety of purposes. Consider the question, 'Can I analyse what I know?'

What you know and can do
You might answer, 'I know how to analyse what I know in that I can:

- compare and contrast the countries of the EC
- distinguish, appraise and debate the principles of management
- analyse, examine and criticise the definition of a contract
- compare different techniques of solving particular types of problems.'

5. Synthesis of knowledge

A still higher level of knowledge may be reflected in the ability to bring together different elements of what you know and present them in a new way, or create a different framework for them to produce a new idea. Consider the question, 'Can I put together elements of knowledge for various fields/sources and arrange them so as to produce a pattern which was not there before?'

What you know and can do
You might answer, 'I can produce new ideas in that I can:

- formulate policies
- propose policies for the future development of the EC
- teach/redesign the principles of management
- develop new ideas about management
- redefine a contract
- suggest modifications to a contract
- develop new ways of solving problems.'

6. Applications of knowledge

Here you are in a position to evaluate or judge material by applying criteria of various kinds to it. Consider the following questions. 'Can I assess the value of what I know?' 'Can I make judgements about what I know?'

What you know and can do
You might answer, 'I can assess what I know in various ways. For example, I can:

- assess the EC in the light of political, social and economic theories
- evaluate/appraise the principles of management
- assess the validity of a contract
- judge the effectiveness of a contract in protecting against business risks
- decide the effectiveness of different approaches to problem solving, both in theory and in practice.'

ACTIVITY: levels of learning

Below are listed six common learning skills:

- organisation of time
- setting personal objectives
- communicating with others through written reports memorandums, etc
- communicating with others orally
- problem solving
- information management.

attended which have not been formally credited. There is also scope to include information on articles you have written, research projects you have undertaken and other work-related experience. You can refer back to this information at any time throughout your profile.

Private record There are some parts of your profile which you will wish to remain confidential. These might include pieces of writing, poems and drawings. You can use this part of your profile to take stock of your past learning, identify your weaknesses, reflect on what you are learning and test out new knowledge.

Competencies, skills and knowledge in respect of award sought (if using the profile for accreditation) This will form the main body of your profile. It needs to include an outline of each of the skills, knowledge and competencies against which you are seeking to be assessed, and a detailed description of what you have learnt, together with evidence to support the learning you have described.

Within most courses, students are expected to produce papers, complete essays, give presentations and write reports. So, too, through your profile you are being asked to demonstrate that you really do possess the knowledge and skills you claim. However, your profile offers you the opportunity to do so in a creative way, which is unique to you. Should you wish to do so, you can include:

- photographs
- articles, poems or short stories you have written
- computer packages you have designed
- care plans you have prepared
- drawings or designs you have undertaken
- reports you have written
- research you have undertaken.

The list is endless. You will also wish to include letters, testimonials and evidence of any public recognition you have received from others. (This might take the form of an article written by someone praising your skill, courage or bravery.)

As you progress, your draft plan will probably change several times in either its organisation or the topics you decide to cover. Continually review your progress and make changes to any draft plan you have made. This will ensure that you achieve a coherent and consistent profile at the end.

Organisation

Your profile has been written to be read and assessed by others. It is more than likely that the person assessing your work does not know you, or has no clear idea as to your academic ability. It is important, therefore, that your profile is easily accessible, clear to read and easy to follow. In your desire to 'tell everything you know', you may forget that someone has to read and make sense of what has been written. The first tip in organising your profile, therefore, is to include features which will help the reader.

Contents page

This should give the reader the main headings in the text, a breakdown of what will be included within each of these, together with clearly marked page numbering.

Cross-reference section

You will probably find that you wish to refer to the same experience to identify a range of competencies or skills. You might also wish to show the same competence or skill at different levels or for different purposes, throughout your profile. Unless you include a competence or skills cross-reference section in your profile, therefore, the reader will find the material confusing. Include this cross-reference section at the beginning of your profile, highlighting areas you have written about or identified throughout your work which you wish the reader to recognise. Your cross-reference page might look like this:

Identification of competencies in being able to work effectively in a multi-disciplinary team:

- Communication skills – pages 10, 15, 34 and 13
- Presentation skills – pages 17, 14 and 13

Introduction

The reader will want to know that your profile is authentic – that it is really your own work. The best way of achieving this is by presenting your profile from a personal as well as professional viewpoint. Introducing the reader to yourself and your aspirations is therefore an essential part of this process. The introduction need not be more than a few sheets of A4. Simply tell the reader why you wish to develop your profile, what your future educational goals and aspirations are, and how you think the assessment of your profile will assist you in achieving your goals. You might wish to include photographs or pictures which illustrate your writing. Remember to state clearly your aims for completing your profile.

Identification of learning

This is the main body of your profile and will be used to demonstrate your relevant skills, knowledge and experience. Within this section you will need to include evidence that you can genuinely do what you claim. The person assessing your profile will be particularly concerned with what you provide as direct evidence of what you know and can do. This should take up the body of the text. However, you will probably wish to have your claims ratified in some way. In this section you can include your references and testimonials.

Other information

Some of the following can be incorporated within the body of the profile or in separate sections:

Appendices These might include testimonials, references and a bibliography of publications.

Samples of work This refers to work which cannot be incorporated within the main body of the text but which enhances what you have written, such as a newspaper article you have written, details of a workshop for which you have been responsible, or details of a campaign you have organised.

Samples from your reflective diary You might also wish to show the extent of your personal and professional development through the process of producing your profile. This would be very useful if you were submitting your profile for professional development purposes. You might include topics you have written about, observations made, reflections upon the profile process, and development of specific skills (e.g. writing).

Sample framework

By now, you should have decided on the structure of your profile and are beginning to work on different aspects of it. The draft for the contents of your profile, therefore, might look like this:

1 **Introduction**
   Introduction about me
   Who I am
   Why I wish to complete a profile
   My experience, goals and education/professional
   aspirations/needs

2 **An introduction to my skills, knowledge and abilities**
   My professional record
      Past jobs
      Past experience
      Qualifications
      Articles written

My private record
Personal knowledge acquired through professional
practice (i.e. committees, organisational
membership outside of work, articles written)

3 **Competencies, skills and knowledge in respect of
award sought**
Communication skills
Skills in critical reflection
Ability to work on own initiative

4 **Indirect evidence**
Testimonials
References

5 **Appendices**

As you progress your draft contents will probably change in
either organisation or topics covered.

Writing skills

Most people, when they begin their profile, are concerned
that they have not written in this way for a long time and are
not good at it. Bear in mind that you are not being asked to
write in exam conditions. With practice, profiling will enable
you to write creatively and effectively in ways that genuinely
reflect what you know, feel and can do. The best place to
practise writing is in your reflective diary. This is because it is
a private place and will allow you to try out new ways of
writing, make mistakes, experiment with new words and
ideas, and discover new ways of organising and presenting
your work. We explore this in more detail in the next chapter.

References

Hull, C. (1993) 'Making Sense of Profiling', in N. Graves (ed) *Learner
Managed Learning: Practice, Theory and Policy*, Higher Education for
Capability: Leeds

Further Education Unit (1987) *Assessing Experiential Learning*, FEU: London

Learning from Experience Trust (1988) *Levels of Learning: A Learners' Introduction to Building on Your Experience*, Learning from Experience Trust: London

Profiles and Reflective Practice 5

The reflective practice movement has been influential in the way profiles are being used within the profession. This chapter explores some of the theories that underpin reflection. It also offers some practical structures that can be used for reflective practice, which will be particularly useful for those who are just beginning.

It would be difficult to write a book about profiles and not include a chapter on reflective practice. Some would argue that the whole purpose of a profile is to develop reflective skills. Whether you agree with this view or not, it is impossible to ignore that being able to reflect on what you do as a professional is becoming increasingly important, and that you are expected to record those reflections in some way – often within a profile or portfolio.

It will not be possible to cover all there is to know about reflective practice in this chapter. Books which explore the subject of reflective practice in greater depth and breadth are listed in the Annotated Bibliography. We aim to give you a working knowledge of what reflective practice is, how it could contribute to improving your practice, how to approach reflective practice as a skill, and how to use your profile to record your reflections.

Reflection and reflective practice are terms that have become increasingly popular and important for many professions, including nursing and midwifery, since the early 1990s. Reflection is becoming recognised by nurses and midwives as an essential component of professional practice, particularly since the popularisation of Schon's book, *The Reflective Practitioner*. Schon (1983) was not the first person to write about reflective practice, nor has he written particularly about health care professionals. However, his work, along with that of Boud *et al* (1985), Dewey (1933) and others, has been influential in the way nursing and midwifery have embraced the subject of reflective practice.

Reflective practice has moved from a passing fancy or 'bandwagon' (as it was described by critics in the early 1990s) to a central theme that runs through most nursing curricula. It is part of the UKCC's standards for post-registration education and practice (PREP), and is central to the nursing policy on clinical supervision. All of this suggests that the reflective practice movement is growing in strength and influence, and can no longer be ignored.

Role of reflection in professional practice

Why is reflective practice important to professional groups and considered to be a part of professional development? Schon (1983) explored the nature of professional practice and tried to explain the role reflection can play in professional action. He recognised that professional work is exceedingly complex and often fast moving, with decisions needing to be made about the best alternatives as you go along.

He suggested that different professions shared common characteristics:

- Professionals face complex problems in their day-to-day work. There are often no definitively right or wrong answers, but only good and not so good ones.
- When making decisions, professionals draw on a knowledge base which is broad, deep and multi-faceted.

- The context in which professionals use their knowledge and skills is very important.
- Professional knowledge is not just about having expert skills.
- It is often difficult for professionals to say or write about what they know and how they use their knowledge.

Clarke, James and Kelly (1994) argue that Schon's real contribution to professionals was to reveal how they cope with these complex problems and what part reflection can play in that.

Schon talks about two types of reflection: reflection-on-action and reflection-in-action. Reflection-on-action occurs when practitioners actively look back and think about an aspect of their practice, and by doing so gain a greater understanding of themselves and the actions and decisions that they took. Reflection-in-action occurs during practice, when practitioners use their learning from previous similar experiences and apply it to their current situation. They are drawing on knowledge they have gained from previous experiences and have internalised, although they may not be able to articulate it at the time. This is sometimes referred to as tacit knowledge. The learning from similar practice situations is used to make sense of what is happening now.

Reflection and learning

As you will have realised from what we have said so far, reflection can lead to learning taking place. If you learn something from reflection, it then gives you an opportunity to use that learning to change your practice or behaviour in some way. The learning can lead to relatively simple changes. For example, you may realise that one way of carrying out a nursing skill is more successful than another; as soon as you have realised that, you can choose to do it in the new way from then on. The learning that occurs can, however, be more complex and personal. For example, you may realise that certain types of patient always seem to annoy you because they remind you of someone in your past.

Figure 5.1   Kolb's learning cycle

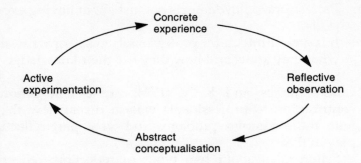

The connection between reflection and learning is often explained by the use of Kolb's learning cycle (see Figure 5.1). You may have already come across this if you have studied the subject of learning from experience (experiential learning). The basic steps are found in other similar models, such as Gibbs' reflective cycle (see Figure 5.2).

These models identify the various stages people pass through when learning from experience and are useful learning tools in themselves. However, they often represent a

Figure 5.2   Gibbs' reflective cycle

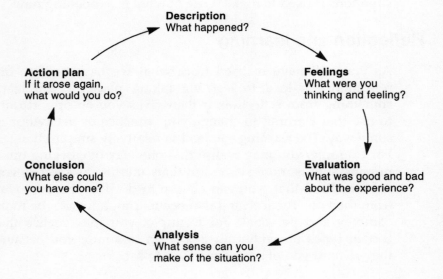

false picture – in the real world, the stages identified in the cycle do not operate as such a smooth process. The diagrams imply that one stage always leads to another, but in reality all experiences are not transformed into general concepts; all concepts are not analysed; and not all concepts are tested out in the world. Sheckley and Keeton (1994) realised that the cycle is subjected to the influence of the person who is trying to learn from his or her experience. They believe that people act as 'information processors' who quickly grasp ideas that confirm personal views and beliefs, but resist and possibly reject ideas that do not confirm existing viewpoints. To illustrate their theory, Sheckley and Keeton have adapted Kolb's learning cycle, as shown in Figure 5.3.

Figure 5.3   Sheckley and Keeton's learning cycle

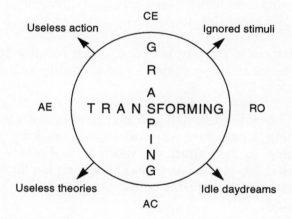

Remember, any model is just a way of representing something – in this case how you can learn from experience. These models provide a theoretical explanation of why it is that you can learn from experience and the part reflection can play in that. If you find them useful, then use them to help others understand. If you find them unhelpful, then there is no need to worry – you do not need to fully understand or accept them to be able to reflect. They may make sense when you feel more comfortable with your reflective skills, and it might be worth looking at the models again at that point.

Defining reflection and reflective practice

There have been many attempts to define reflective practice. Some definitions are more helpful than others; have a look at the following popularly quoted ones and decide which makes most sense to you.

Reflective practice can be interpreted as being the practitioner's ability to access, make sense of and learn through work experience to achieve more desirable, effective and satisfying work. (Johns, 1995)

The process of internally examining and exploring an issue of concern, triggered by an experience, which creates and clarifies meaning in terms of self, and which results in a changed conceptual perspective.
(Boyd and Fales, 1983)

Systematic enquiry into one's own practice to improve practice and deepen one's understanding of it.
(Lucas, 1991)

These definitions tell you that reflection is about thinking, learning from your experience and making use of that learning in the future. If you are to become a reflective practitioner, you have to use that learning to expand your professional knowledge to the benefit of your patients, and yourself.

Whilst reflection and some of the theories that lie behind it are relatively new, thinking about what you have done in your professional practice is not. When nurses and midwives first start to read about reflection and reflective practice, they often say, 'but we are already doing this; what's new about this?' Of course, in talking about reflective practice no one is suggesting that nurses and midwives have not thought about their practice before. Schon, by describing how professionals behave, was not inventing a new way of behaving; he was uncovering and exposing behaviours that had gone on before, and trying to make sense of them by giving them a structure and framework. He wrote about this so that others could benefit from what he had found.

Reflection is a process which allows you to uncover and expose actions, thoughts, feelings and behaviours which are present during a period of time. You can use this process to look at any aspect of your life where you want to understand more about what you do and how you can develop. Through understanding more about your professional practice – why you use certain interventions and in what situations – you can extend your personal professional knowledge beyond that found in text books or published research. It is this potential to extend professional knowledge which makes the process of reflection much more than just thinking about practice.

Reflection and profiles

Most of the commercially available profiles address the issue of reflection and reflective practice. At its simplest, a profile provides a storage place for some of the written outcomes of reflection. But many profiles do much more than that by encouraging and explaining the skills of reflection. For example, the Nursing Times (now Macmillan Open Learning) *Profile Pack* encourages you to keep a reflective diary. The authors believe that a continuous process of reflection is an effective way of developing personally and professionally because it can help you to:

- understand the complexity of your work
- analyse your experience and view it more critically
- value your experience
- develop a sense of ownership of your professional development
- confront and think through 'upsetting' incidents
- create an agenda for discussion with others
- appreciate your own development by seeing changes over time, which can lead to an increase in confidence.

The English National Board *Professional Portfolio* also

encourages reflection in relation to the ten key characteristics of professional practice (see Chapter 1). It encourages you to reflect in this more structured way so that you can demonstrate learning outcomes in relation to the ENB continuing professional education framework.

If you are following a particular study programme, it is becoming increasingly likely that there will be requirements for you to maintain a profile and (or within it) a reflective diary. Sections of this diary may form part of the assessment scheme for the programme and this should be made clear to you at the outset. The diary's contribution to the assessment scheme may be about demonstrating your reflective skills, or it may be about demonstrating how you are using the outcomes of your reflections in practice.

The implementation of PREP now requires you to maintain a Personal Professional Profile throughout your career. For this, the development of reflective practice skills will be helpful. UKCC Fact Sheet 4 explains that the profile document is more than a record of achievement. It encourages you to use the profile document as a continuous process which involves 'reflecting and recording what you learn from everyday experiences'.

The UKCC believes that profiling is a continuous process which breaks down into three steps:

- Step 1 is about reviewing your experience to date.
- Step 2 is about self-appraisal.
- Step 3 is about setting goals and action planning.

Self-appraisal (step 2) relies heavily on the concept of reflection-on-action, and Fact Sheet 4 gives a brief framework of questions that you can use to reflect on a particular aspect of your practice. When thinking about the UKCC requirements for profiling and reflection, it will be important to refer to this fact sheet. It gives you information about the minimum amount of this type of activity you will need to record in order to successfully re-register.

The UKCC will randomly audit a sample of registrants each year to ensure its requirements are being met. Self-appraisal of professional performance is one of the areas where it may request information about your:

- strengths and weaknesses
- achievements
- analysis of significant events through reflection-on-action
- development needs.

Writing and reflecting

The process of reflection does not have to be written down. It is possible to reflect inside your head, rather like doing mental arithmetic. However, our experience has shown that more insights are gained if writing is involved.

The action of writing is useful for several reasons:

- It means that you get the thoughts out of your head and onto paper, where they can be examined and analysed in a less personal and more objective way.
- The process of constructing words and sentences gives structure to your thoughts and recollections.
- A written account gives you a permanent record, which you can read immediately or at a later date to gain further insights.
- If you write on a regular basis and record significant events at the time they happen, this will provide an accurate record to work with.

The whole point of reflective practice (which includes writing things down) is so that you can learn from your professional practice. Walker (1985) has devised, through the experience of working with students, some useful tips on gaining the most from your reflective writing:

- Be frank and honest in your entries. Write it as it is, not as you would like it to be. Be open and sincere in what you record.
- Have a positive approach to the profile. Recognise the

potential that it has, and approach it as something that can give you things in return.

- Be spontaneous. Do not spend a lot of time working out what you are going to write, just get something down on paper. It is very useful simply to write and then reflect on what is written

- Feel free to express yourself in your profile in ways other than writing. Use diagrams, pictures, drawings and other types of material. Sometimes a picture can express what you are trying to say more effectively.

- The profile is meant to be a workbook. Use underlining, circling or highlighter pens to draw out things of significance. As your profile builds up, it is important to go back to the early entries and to reflect further on them.

- Be spontaneous – use your own words to express what you are thinking, feeling and realising. You are not writing an essay that will be marked or making an entry for the Booker prize, so do not worry about the way that you write.

- Be prepared to change your style of working with the profile. Feel free to try different methods – discover your own style.

- Take up the issues that surface when you are working with the profile. Do not get distracted by other more trivial things.

- Persevere in the face of initial difficulties; be faithful to it.

Confidentiality

As we are encouraging you to write down information about yourself and your patients and colleagues, it is important that we address the issue of confidentiality. There are two aspects to consider when considering confidentiality: how to protect your patients and colleagues, and how to protect yourself.

As Walker suggests, it is important that your writings are honest and spontaneous. Whilst writing reflectively, you should not have to be concerned about who might read it. If you are, you may start to censor what you are writing to avoid offending the people concerned, or make any feelings you express suitable for public consumption. If you take this approach, because you are concerned people will read your profile, it is likely to reduce what you gain personally from the writing process.

It is important to remember that no one has the right to read your profile without your permission. The UKCC reminds registrants that 'your profile contains confidential information about you and should, therefore, not be accessible to others without your permission'.

When deciding whether to give your permission, you need to understand their reason for wanting to read it. Knowing the reason behind the request will enable you to select parts of your profile that are relevant to their interest.

For example, in Fact Sheet 4 the UKCC specifies which parts of your profile it may request to see at the point of you re-registering. It is making it clear in advance of a possible request, so that you can organise your profile accordingly and screen out any aspects that are not of interest to the UKCC or areas that you would not wish to disclose. The UKCC (1995) suggests that you might consider dividing your profile into two parts: one that contains strictly confidential information; the other that contains information which the UKCC may require for audit purposes.

It is now quite common for students completing pre- and post-registration programmes to be asked to keep reflective diaries as part of the programme, sometimes as part of the assessment scheme. These reflective diaries can be part of a profile or asked for as a stand-alone item. The programme organisers should make this clear at the outset and you should be clear what is going to happen to any parts of the diary that have to be given in during the programme. Will it be assessed? If so, what are the criteria for assessment? How many people will see your diary entries? How will they be stored? Will they be copied? Will the copies and the original be returned to you in the future?

When writing about patients and colleagues, it is best not to identify them by name. In Fact Sheet 4 the UKCC advises that 'you do not document any information which could in any way identify patients, clients or carers, as this could constitute a breach of confidentiality'.

It is also important that writings within a reflective diary are not taken out of context, particularly if you are really trying to be open and honest in your reflections. For example, you may have written about a colleague who had made you really angry, and the expression of your anger has been full and free in your diary entry. Having expressed the anger and worked it through, you learn something new about yourself and realise that the colleague was not the one responsible for your anger. Anyone reading your diary entry who did not understand the whole context of the situation, including what you had learnt from it, may well be left with the impression that you do not get on with that colleague. An understanding of the context of reflective writings is essential, and you should consider this when deciding what to disclose to whom.

Reflection – how do you do it?

Learning to reflect and learning from those reflections is a very individual process. There are many useful structures available – examples by Johns (1995) and Stephenson (1994) are outlined below – but, according to L'Aiguille (1994), reflection can only be learnt by having a go. Some people are more naturally reflective than others, but reflection is a skill that can be learnt, practised and refined by anyone.

In the following section we are going to provide guidance on reflection for those who have no or very little experience of the subject. It is much easier, when starting out, to grasp the skills of reflecting on situations from the past – what Schon (1983) called reflection-on-action. The five main steps to the reflective process are:

1   set aside time to reflect in a place where there will be no distractions
2   choose a situation or event to reflect upon
3   critically reflect on the situation or event

4   identify areas of learning and decide on any necessary
     follow-up actions
5   revisit and re-evaluate.

We will now look at each of these in more detail.

Step 1   Set aside time to reflect in a place where there will be no distractions

Find a place which is comfortable and private, with no
distractions. You will need writing materials. At first you
might find that any piece of paper will do, but if you are
going to keep a reflective diary on a regular basis, then buy a
book to write in so that everything can be kept together.

It may take some time to work through the steps in the
process, so you will need to set aside at least 2–3 hours. You
can break off between the steps and return if you want, but
this is easier to do once you become more familiar and
comfortable with reflection.

If you speak to colleagues who are already using reflective
skills, you will probably find they have a special place, book
design or pen they use when making entries in their
reflective diaries. This may sound strange and unnecessary,
and to some extent it is, but making the process special in
some way shows how they value it – and, in turn, how they
value themselves. Keeping a reflective diary needs a lot of
motivation and commitment, and some people find it easier
than others. Find out over a period of time and through
experimentation what works best for you. If that means
writing with a special pen or in a special place, use it!

Step 2   Choose a situation or event to reflect upon

Most people start by reflecting on a situation from their area
of practice. It does not matter how you choose the situation –
trust your instincts. If a situation pops into your head for no
apparent reason, then do not reject it, choose to work with it.
You may have heard that people are asked to reflect on
'critical incidents' and worry that the situation you have

thought of is not *critical* enough. People's interpretation of 'critical' is often influenced by the medical use of the word, meaning seriously ill. The situation you choose to work with does not have to be like this. It can be a routine and outwardly mundane situation that you meet every day and are very familiar with. On the other hand, it might be a situation that sticks in your mind for some other reason. The point we are making here is that the situation you choose to reflect on just has to mean something and be significant to *you*.

Critical incident technique was originated by Flanagan – an aviation psychologist – during the Second World War, when the US Air Force needed to select and train air crews as effectively as possible. He defined an incident as 'any observable activity that is sufficiently complete in itself to permit inferences and predictions about the person performing the act'. Flanagan was using critical incidents to observe others, whereas you are using his ideas to observe yourself.

So, having chosen a critical incident or situation to reflect on, what do you do next? You need to recall the details of the situation in your mind's eye and then write about it. Some people find it easier to close their eyes to recall the situation and to replay the scene in their mind, rather like rerunning a video of the event. It is important that you recall as many details as possible, such as:

- where the event took place
- who was involved
- what actually happened
- how you were involved
- what your feelings were at the time
- what contribution you made to the situation
- what the consequences of that were
- what happened after the situation.

All of this detail needs to be written down, in whatever way makes sense to you. Remember, the writing is for you to work with, not for someone to mark. You can write in any style and in any way that you find comfortable. The important thing is to try and include as much detail as possible. You are likely to find that writing about one aspect of the event triggers memories of other aspects that you have forgotten. It may also trigger connections with other memories; these connections are important, however disconnected they may seem on the surface, so write them down too.

Some people find they want to draw diagrams or pictures to illustrate the situation, they are reflecting on. Do not feel restrained by our initial advice to write about the situation – if you want to draw, then feel free to.

Recalling the situation in the way we have described allows you to stand back and 'observe' the event as it happened. The distance encourages you to be objective.

In recalling the situation you might record the feelings that were present at the time. You might just write about them – 'I felt really pleased with myself' or 'I felt really annoyed' – or, as you are writing about the feelings, you may actually re-experience them. There may be a mixture of positive and negative feelings. The feelings you experience need to be acknowledged by you, so they do not become a barrier to you progressing with the reflective process.

Step 3   Critically reflect on the situation or event

Just recreating a situation from your nursing past, however, is not enough on its own. Once you have recalled it, you need to do something with it. Remember that the whole purpose of reflection is to learn something from it and extend your personal practice knowledge base.

Structures for reflection

How can you critically reflect on your actions from the past? It is useful to use some type of structure for this. You may want to create your own structure, but being a beginner it may be useful to use one of the structures that already exist within the literature. Many of the frameworks in the literature are composed of a series of questions to ask yourself once you have recalled the situation you are going to reflect upon. These structures have been devised by people who have had a great deal of experience with reflection and it seems foolish not to benefit from that experience, certainly in the first instance. As you become more confident, you can adjust, adapt and refine their structures to make them more personal and relevant to you.

We are including two structures for critical reflection here. References for others are included in the Annotated Bibliography.

Holm and Stephenson (1994)
This first structure was developed by Debi Holm and Sarah Stephenson, two students who were immersed in reflection over a four-year period. They suggest that once you have recalled a situation, you should ask yourself the following questions.

- What was my role in this situation?
- Did I feel comfortable or uncomfortable? Why?
- What actions did I take?
- How did I and others act?
- Was it appropriate?
- How could I have improved the situation for myself, the patient, my mentor?
- What can I change in the future?
- Do I feel as if I have learnt anything new about myself?
- Did I expect anything different to happen? What and why?
- Has it changed my way of thinking in any way?
- What knowledge from theory and research can I apply to this situation ?
- What broader issues, for example ethical, political or social, arise from this situation?
- What do I think about these broader issues?

Johns (1994)
This second structure was devised by Chris Johns, who has experience as a researcher, teacher and facilitator of the

reflective process. He calls it a 'model of structured reflection'. As well as asking questions about feelings, it also considers the background to the experience and factors which influenced the way you acted. Another feature of this model is that it asks you to think about alternative choices you could have made, and the implications of the experience for your own learning.

For the questions about learning, Johns has been influenced by the work of Carper (1978). This suggests there are four distinct areas of knowledge needed by nurses and midwives:

- empirics
- aesthetics
- ethics
- personal.

Empirics refers to the science of nursing; aesthetics is the art of nursing; ethics is the moral component; and personal refers to the personal relationship which exists between nurse and patient. These are sometimes referred to as Carper's four 'patterns of knowing'.

Model of structured reflection
Core question: What information do I need access to in order to learn through this experience?

Cue questions
1.0 *Description of the experience*
1.1 Phenomenon – Describe the 'here and now' experience
1.2 Causal – What essential factors contributed to this experience?
1.3 Context – What are the significant background factors to this experience?
1.4 Clarifying – What are the key processes (for reflection) in this experience?

2.0 *Reflection*
2.1 What was I trying to achieve?

2.2 Why did I intervene as I did?

2.3 What were the consequences of my actions for:
- myself
- the patient/family
- the people I work with?

2.4 How did I feel about this experience when it was happening?

2.5 How did the patient feel about it?

2.6 How did I know how the patient felt about it?

3.0 *Influencing factors*

3.1 What internal factors influenced my decision making?

3.2 What external factors influenced my decision making?

3.3 What sources of knowledge did/should have influenced my decision making?

4.0 *Could I have dealt better with the situation?*

4.1 What other choices did I have?

4.2 What would be the consequences of these choices?

5.0 *Learning*

5.1 How do I now feel about this experience?

5.2 How have I made sense of this experience in light of past experiences and future practices?

5.3 How has this experience changed my ways of knowing?
- empirics (what does it tell me about the science of nursing?)
- aesthetics (what does it tell me about the art of nursing?)
- ethics (what does it add to my understanding of moral issues?)
- personal (what does it add to my understanding of myself and my relationships with patients?)

Johns is constantly refining this structure in the light of his experience with students and practitioners. If you find the whole model too daunting and theoretical at first, then use the parts of it you feel most comfortable with.

Individual or group work

You can choose whether to use a structure on your own, with a trusted friend or friends, or in a reflective practice group facilitated by a suitably experienced person.

Johns (1994) argues strongly for the benefits of reflecting in a group or with the support of a facilitator, rather than on your own. His work and research show that reflecting can be very difficult to do without expert guidance and support. Being in a group should be supportive, and you can often learn as much from the reflections of others as you can from your own. The group is also likely to be facilitated by a skilled person who can help and guide you with the reflective process.

In addition, a group situation brings the opportunity for supportive challenge from other group members, which prevents you being unrealistic in the conclusions you draw from your reflections. In other words, the group gives you the chance to check whether your perceptions of yourself and the way you acted in a situation are the same as their perceptions. Whilst there are no right or wrongs here, alternative viewpoints can provide learning opportunities.

Whilst supporting the view that an expert facilitator can bring a different approach to reflection, not everyone has access to such a facilitator or group. To meet the UKCC requirement, all practitioners will have to learn the basic skills of reflection, using the self-appraisal questions outlined in Fact Sheet 4 (UKCC, 1995).

Step 4 Identify areas of learning and decide on any necessary follow-up actions.

This step is crucial in the reflective process and yet a lot of people fail to 'convert' their reflections into learning. It forms the major difference between genuine reflection and what nurses have always done when thinking about their practice. At this stage, you should actually begin to identify what you have learnt from reflecting on a critical incident, or what you need to learn before participating in this type of care again. It is important to learn from your successes as well as your difficulties. What worked well in a situation? Does that type of approach/intervention always work well? Is it possible to generalise from this situation to others?

Compare what you have learnt from your own practice with information from other professionals and the literature. See if what you have discovered through reflection is borne out by the theories, techniques and research of others. This fits very well with the Lucas (1991) definition of reflection, which talks about 'systematic enquiry into one's own practice to improve that practice and deepen one's understanding of it'.

If your learning from reflection – which makes up your own personal professional knowledge base – is borne out by others, then this can be helpful as it gives your learning a professional (contextual) validity. If the literature does not support what you have found, this does not mean you are wrong. It may give you ideas to investigate the subject further when you have the opportunity. A literature search may reveal insights or solutions to situations that you would like to improve or change.

Step 5   Revisit and re-evaluate

It is helpful to revisit your reflections from time to time. Of course, this comment assumes that you are keeping a record – written or otherwise – of your reflections and any follow-up actions you decide to take. Revisiting these records is helpful for a number of reasons:

- It can help you realise how far you have travelled since you started to reflect (or from the last time you revisited your journal). It is always satisfying to see your own progress.
- It can help you to identify any patterns in the things you have been working with through the reflective process. For example, do the critical incidents always involve communication difficulties, or difficulties with a particular technique? Does this pattern tell you anything about an area of continuing education you may need to follow?

Ideas for further work on reflection

As we said at the beginning, there is much more to reflection than this chapter can cover. The art and science of reflection is being refined all the time as more people work with it, write about it and share their experiences.

There are several things you can choose to reflect on when you become more confident with the skills, such as:

- major trends in your career, and whether you are satisfied about the way things have gone
- the way you interact with other members of the multi-professional team, and what contribution you make
- how you deal with constructive criticism and feedback from peers
- how you have coped with challenges and dealt with areas of your practice that need improvement
- how you have made the best use of your talents, qualities and strengths.

These examples can be very challenging at first, because they explore personal issues about who you are and how you respond. However, we encourage you to try out some of the ideas once you feel more confident.

References

Boud, D., Keogh, R. and Walker, D. (1985) *Reflection: Turning Experience into Learning*, Kogan Page: London

Boyd, E. M. and Fales, A. W. (1983) 'Reflecting Learning: Key to Learning from Experience', *Journal of Humanistic Psychology*, 23, 2, 99–117

Carper, B. (1978) 'Fundamental Ways of Knowing in Nursing', *Advances in Nursing Science*, 11, 13–23

Clarke, B., James, C. R. and Kelly, J. (1994) 'Reflective Practice: Reviewing the Issues and Refocusing the Debate', unpublished paper given at the 1994 Macmillan Open Learning Conference on Clinical Nurse Specialists, Nottingham

Dewey, J. (1933) *How We Think*, DC Health and Co: Boston

ENB (1991) *Professional Portfolio*, ENB Publications: London

Flanagan, J. C. (1954) 'The Critical Incident Technique', *Psychological Bulletin*, 5, 327–58

Gibbs, G. (1988) *Learning By Doing: A Guide to Teaching and Learning Methods*, Further Education Unit, Oxford Polytechnic: Oxford

Johns, C. (1995) 'The Value of Reflective Practice for Nursing', *Journal of Clinical Nursing*, 4, 23–40

Kolb, D. (1984) *Experiential Learning: Experience as a Source of Learning and Development*, Prentice Hall: New Jersey

L'Aiguille, Y. (1994) in A. Palmer, S. Burns and C. Bulman *Reflective Practice in Nursing – The Growth of the Professional Practitioner*, Blackwell Scientific: Oxford

Lucas, P. (1991) 'Reflection, New Practices and the need for Flexibility in Supervising Student Teachers', *Journal of Further and Higher Education*, 15, 2, 84–93

Mezirow, J. (1981) 'A Critical Theory of Adult Learning and Education', in M. Tight (ed) *Learning and Education*, Croom Helm: Kent

Palmer, A., Burns S., and Bulman, C. (eds) *Reflective Practice in Nursing: The Growth of the Professional Practitioner*, Blackwell Scientific: Oxford

Schon, D. (1983) *The Reflective Practitioner*, Basic Books Inc: New York

Sheckley, B. and Keeton, M. (1994) 'Learning From Experience' unpublished paper given at 1994 International Experiential Learning Conference, Washington USA

Stephenson, S. (1994) in A. Palmer, S. Burns and C. Bulman *Reflective Practice in Nursing: The Growth of the Professional Practitioner*, Blackwell Scientific: Oxford

UKCC (1995) 'UKCC's Standards for Post Registration Education and Practice (PREP)', *Fact Sheets 1–8*, UKCC: London

Walker, D. (1985) in D. Baud, R. Keogh and D. Walker *Reflection: Turning Experience into Learning*, Kogan Page: London

Making Your Learning Count 6

The profile you develop will largely be determined by the
system through which you are seeking accreditation. In this
chapter, therefore, we begin by exploring the concept of
accreditation as it is currently used within professional
education, and we suggest a working definition. We then
move on to look at the implications this has for your own
working practices. In this chapter we explore the meanings
behind the following terms in depth: Credit Accumulation
and Transfer Scheme (CATS); National Vocational Qualifications (NVQs); assessment of prior learning (APL); assessment
of prior experiential learning (APEL).

Since the mid 1980s there has been an increasing awareness,
within both the public and private sector, of the need for
practitioners to develop skills and knowledge which will
allow them to maintain professional competence throughout
their working lives. This, in turn, has meant finding ways of
giving formal recognition to what is already known and can
be done, regardless of whether this knowledge has been
achieved through formal courses of study or informally and
through life experience. One reason for this is that, in
forecasts for the year 2000, employers have consistently
stressed that:

- of all new jobs in the UK, 90 per cent will require graduate ability and above
- 70 per cent of all jobs in Europe will require high-level vocational skills.

Significantly, what is required is not an educated elite. Rather, the skills and knowledge of workers at all levels must be raised. As five out of six people in the workforce of the year 2000 are already in work, this means that upgrading Britain's current workforce will require a massive effort. The legacy of the past has left Britain's current workforce with lower levels of basic attainment, fewer qualifications, and narrower skills than in Germany, France or Japan.

Clearly this has contributed to the current interest in the development of giving recognition to formal and informal learning, within both public and private sector professions. In education and training it has meant that increasing emphasis is being given to developing more flexible approaches to learning. A flexible education system is one that is geared up to meet the needs of the student, rather than the organisation. A flexible system should allow people to have greater control over their own learning. This includes more choice about content and method of assessment, as well as the preferred time and location of learning.

All of this is important for several reasons. Firstly, it means that you no longer have to give up work in order to study for a substantial qualification such as a degree or professional award. Secondly, you do not have to learn what you already know and can do, so your learning can become more challenging and relevant. Thirdly it allows your learning to be recognised wherever and however it has occurred, such as through open or distance learning, formal courses, or through life and work experiences. Finally, it means that you are now better able to plan your learning to fit in with existing work and family commitments.

The emphasis on flexible learning has, in turn, created a need to develop more flexible approaches to the process of accrediting learning. Before we examine some of these flexible frameworks for credit, we need to clarify what we understand by the term accreditation.

Towards a definition of accreditation

A simple definition of accreditation is that it is the process of giving formal recognition or validation to skills, knowledge, experience or competence. In short, it is giving public recognition to what you already know and can demonstrate. However, the term accreditation is also used to apply to an organisation or institution's ability to uphold specific standards, and to the process of approving awards. In the broadest sense then, the term accreditation can be used to describe the assessment and certification arrangements for particular programmes of study and awards, as well as the outcome for you as a learner.

Within any definition of accreditation is also the recognition that the process includes interpretation. So, submitting your learning for credit suggests that there is a decision making process regarding what evidence should be caught in assessment and what information recorded in certification.

Recognition of skills, competence or knowledge is not merely a passive or dispassionate acknowledgement that they have been attained. It implies an evaluative judgement about their worth – crudely, a granting of market value. The process of consideration of this market value often relates to what the trainer, teacher or supervisor decides to record on the final certificate. This act of interpretation by the receiving party is as much a part of accreditation as the processes which go into creating those statements. (FESC, 1989)

It might be useful at this point to remind you that although assessment and accreditation are closely connected, they are not the same. Whilst learning cannot be accredited without being assessed, clearly learning can be assessed without being accredited.

Accreditation of continuing professional development

We will now move on to look at some of the current systems available for accrediting prior experiential learning (APEL).

Traditionally, there have been two routes for awarding academic credit. The first was through an individual university establishing its own standards, practices and procedures in order to award its own credit. This route continues to exist. The second route was through a centralised awarding body, called the Council For National Academic Awards (CNAA). This body was largely responsible for monitoring standards, practices and procedures and conferring CNAA status to polytechnics and other colleges of higher education. However, in 1992 the 'binary line' was removed, which meant that polytechnics were given university status. University status means that these 'new universities' are now able to establish their own standards, practices and procedures and award their own academic credit. Because of this, in 1992 CNAA ceased to exist. However, a new unit has now been established to assess and monitor the quality and practices of all universities, old and new.

Continuing professional development (CPD) is the term most commonly associated with the ongoing learning that you need to undertake throughout your career in order to maintain professional knowledge and skills. Many influential bodies, including the English National Board (ENB) and the Central Council For The Education and Training of Social Workers (CCETSW), are now able to award academic credit for professional qualifications and continuing professional development. This is largely because of two nationally recognised flexible accreditation schemes. The first of these is the Credit Accumulation and Transfer Scheme (CATS); the second is National Vocational Qualifications (NVQs). We shall now move on to look at the principles and practices behind each of these schemes.

Credit Accumulation and Transfer Scheme (CATS)

In a report to the DES in 1979, Peter Toyne described CATS as:

> essentially a process whereby qualifications, part qualifications and learning experiences are given appropriate recognition or credit to enable students to progress in their studies without necessarily having to repeat materials or levels of study. (Toyne, 1979)

So, CATS was initially conceived as a means of recruiting students who might not otherwise benefit from higher education, to compensate for the expected fall in the 18-year-old population in the 1990s.

CATS was originally established by the Council For National Academic Awards (CNAA). Although the principles for the scheme and the credit tariff established by the CNAA have largely been adopted by universities and colleges of higher education, this has always been at the discretion of each university.

> The term 'CATS' needs to be defined in order to differentiate between various CATS arrangements. Currently the term is applied to small departmental prototypes, large, institution wide programmes and national consortia arrangements. In other schemes, the focus may be upon part-time learners, individual learning programmes, prior learning, work based learning or professional and in-company training. (HEQC, 1994)

Each institution designs and operates its own CAT scheme and, in some cases, a different credit tariff is offered. Also, because of the Scottish system for higher education, Scotland has developed a unique CAT scheme called SCOTCAT.

CATS and the accreditation of prior experiential learning (APEL)

CATS is based on the principle that appropriate learning, wherever it occurs and provided that it can be assessed, should be given academic credit. This means that people can gain credit for learning they acquire at work, for short courses they have attended, and through life experiences such as bringing up children, voluntary work, unemployment and redundancy. In short, it has provided a system for accrediting prior experiential learning. Having said this, it is important to remember that CATS provides an alternative means of obtaining existing awards and is not a separate series of qualifications.

There are two important principles embedded within CATS. Firstly, credits can be given for prior experiential learning prior to registration with a university for a programme. In other words, you can use your prior experiential learning to gain access to courses or to join a course with advanced standing. Secondly, credits can be obtained through learning from a wide range of institutions and locations other than higher education, such as work-related learning.

A significant aspect of the scheme is therefore the flexibility it allows in the mode of attendance and the locations of study. You can now study either full- or part-time, by open learning or a combination of all of these modes. It also means that if you move from one geographical area to another, you can transfer credit from one institution to another. Neither is credit lost if you have a break in your studies.

The credit tariff scheme is based on two benchmarks:

1 to obtain an Honours degree you must accumulate 360 credit points
2 to obtain a Master's degree you must accumulate 120 credit points at postgraduate level.

In each case the credit points represent the total workload required to obtain the award. Intermediate awards are available at both undergraduate and postgraduate level.

Finally, it is important to understand that a distinction is made between general and specific credit. Learning becomes specific credit when you seek to apply your prior credit to a specific programme of studies for a future award. This means that specific credit refers to the use of general credit within your chosen programme of study.

Professional bodies and CATS

Traditionally distinctions have been made between academic and professional education, formal and informal learning, and vocational and non-vocational education. The CAT scheme, however, places the emphasis on what has been learnt rather than where or how that learning has been acquired. This is clearly good news for professional practice. The CAT scheme provides a framework in which different sectors, institutions and interests are able to break down their professional barriers and find ways of sharing a common dialogue for validating professional learning.

National Vocational Qualifications (NVQs)

During the 1980s, there was growing concern about the lack of vocationally related education and training offered to people both inside and outside work. It was because of this that a wide range of national schemes and programmes, aimed at improving and extending vocational education and training, was established.

With all this in mind, the National Council for Vocational Qualifications (NCVQ) was established in 1986. NCVQ is an independent body, funded by the Government. It has no legal powers and, like CATS, can only effect change with the cooperation of the awarding bodies, industry bodies, professional bodies, and further and higher education. It relies on the Government to use its influence to support the introduction of NVQs. NVQs are qualifications about work. They are based upon standards of competence set by industry. Because they are competence based, it is meeting the standard that is important. So long as you are able to demonstrate that you have met the standard, you can expect to get the credit: 'It is up to individuals how and where they learn – at work, at college or in their own time. There are no barriers. Access to NVQ assessment is open to all. There are no discriminatory rules nor age limits' (Jessup, 1991).

Whereas in CAT schemes learning is defined by learning outcomes, in NVQs learning is defined in terms of competence in specified performance. Being competent is not seen as referring to a low or minimum level of performance. 'On the contrary, it refers to the standard required successfully to perform an activity or function. Being competent means performing to professional or occupational standards. In most professional and occupational areas there is no scope for second best standards' (Jessup, 1991).

Each NVQ is given a title and a level to locate it in the NVQ framework. The NVQ framework is a way of showing how qualifications relate to each other and how you can progress through the system. There are five levels in the framework, level 1 being the most basic.

The framework allows transfer and progression both within occupational areas and between them. This is achieved by grouping together those qualifications that are similar in their statement of competence.

NCVQ argue that this competence-based approach offers:

- sets of competencies (units, elements and performance criteria) derived from analysis of occupational roles
- an assessment process by which performance is matched against the elements and the criteria
- credit for units of competence fulfilled
- an indication of areas in which competence is yet to be achieved.

General National Vocational Qualifications (GNVQs)

As NVQs became established, NCVQ began to look at ways of giving credit for the skills, knowledge and understanding that underpin a range of NVQs within a broad occupational area. In 1992 they introduced General National Vocational

Qualifications (GNVQs). GNVQs are distinct from NVQs in that they are not based upon competence but rather upon a statement of attainment. This means that, in addition to the assessment criteria which apply to NVQs, these new qualifications require you to 'demonstrate an understanding of the principles which underlie the activities specified in general NVQ elements' (Jessup, 1991). In this way GNVQs are comparable in their demands to academic qualifications, whilst also having clear and explicit links with occupational NVQs.

Claiming credit for your prior learning

There are four stages involved in preparing your informal learning to submit for academic or professional credit. These stages are very similar to the process of constructing your profile (see Chapter 4).

- Stage 1: Systematic reflection on experience
- Stage 2: Identification of significant learning
- Stage 3: Identification of evidence to support claims
- Stage 4: Submission of profile for formal assessment

Let us look at each of these stages a little more closely.

Stage 1: Systematic reflection on experience

As you have already seen, reflection is an important part of the APEL process. There are two ways in which you can reflect upon past experiences: you can do it close to the time of the event, or you can reflect some time later. Although you are not always aware, some of your most significant learning experiences might have happened a long time ago, perhaps even in your childhood. The first stage in the APEL process therefore lies in systematically reflecting on experience, in order to identify where significant learning has occurred.

At this stage you are simply being asked to recall your experience. The question you are being asked to address is simply: 'What experiences have I had?' Some people find it useful to 'brainstorm' or talk this through with colleagues and friends. Others find it useful to write a personal biography which includes jobs done, people encountered and places visited. This will depend upon the amount of time you have allotted.

This stage is perhaps the most important one in the process because it will provide you with the substance from which you will be working.

Stage 2: Identification of significant learning

Having mapped out your experience in some form, the next stage is to identify what you have learnt from it. This means focusing on the experiences identified in Stage 1, in order to begin making claims about what you have learnt. Often learning claims are offered as learning statements. You will find more about writing learning claims in Chapter 4. Learning claims normally have two elements to them. Firstly, there is a claim to your knowledge at some level. Secondly, you are making a claim to be able to perform a skill, or to do something. The form in which you present your claims will depend very much on what you are seeking your learning to be assessed against.

Stage 3: Identification of evidence to support claims

One of the purposes in producing a profile is to provide evidence that you have acquired the learning you have described. It is accepted that students in a classroom must provide evidence of their learning in the form of essays, oral presentations or written examinations. Similarly, in the profile process you will be expected to demonstrate that you possess the knowledge or skills you are claiming. What counts as evidence will again depend on the nature of what you are seeking your learning to be assessed against. For example, someone making a claim for credit against a music course might substantiate the claim by writing and playing a music score. A claim to knowledge in computing might be accompanied by a computer package. If you are working in the area of mental health, your claim might point to an education programme you have devised. So, evidence may take many forms. Broadly, there are two types of evidence: direct and indirect.

Direct evidence

This refers to evidence you have directly created. It might include performance you have given, reports you have written, the assessment of your clinical practice or work-based experience. In most cases, direct evidence is the most effective in demonstrating that you really do know and can do what you are claiming. Direct evidence can include a wide range of material, such as:

- a report you have compiled and written (in whole or part)
- an article you have written
- the design of a curriculum
- presentations, speeches, talks or training events you have carried out (this can be managed through an audio or audio-visual tape)
- manuals you have written or designed
- photographs
- drawings, graphs, paintings and sculptures you have made.

This list is not exhaustive and you might think of other things which could be included. However, in all forms of direct evidence you need to show that the work really is yours, or demonstrate the part you played in its development.

Indirect evidence

This refers to evidence from others about your claim to learning. It can take the form of:

- a testimonial from someone with expertise in the field, including a supervisor or manager

- letters written on your behalf by colleagues, including a supervisor or manager; a letter might also come from a professional association or an organisation with whom you have carried out voluntary work
- awards you have received
- magazine, journal or newspaper articles about you
- certificates of attendance at courses and workshops.

Avoid evidence which might suggest bias, such as a letter from a family member or close friend. Also avoid letters or articles about events in which you were involved, but which do not mention you specifically or fail to highlight what you did and the skills you used.

Finally, any evidence you offer should be clearly associated with the particular learning claim. So, for example, if you are approaching a colleague for a reference, s/he will need to be briefed as to the specific learning claim you are seeking to address. Without a link being made between the claim and the evidence, it is difficult to give a realistic assessment of what has been learnt.

Summary of assessment

Your completed profile will include both direct and indirect evidence. Within this you should try to include:

- accounts of relevant experience
- relevant certificates/awards
- supporting documentation
- current assessments
- details of an oral assessment.

Stage 4: Submission of profile for formal assessment

Once you have identified your sources of evidence, you need to prepare your profile for submission. Much of the work will already have been done by this stage; your task now is to assemble it, making it accurate and easy to read. How the profile is submitted will depend largely on the requirements of the validating and accrediting body. We discuss this process and offer practical advice in Chapter 4. Although professionals disagree as to what should be included in a profile and the format it should take, the one thing they all agree upon is the criteria by which it will be finally assessed. These are as follows:

Breadth   The learning is not isolated from wider considerations.

Authenticity   You can do what is claimed.

Quality   The learning is at the appropriate academic level.

Currency   You have kept up to date with recent developments.

Acceptability   The evidence supports the learning claim to which it is linked.

Sufficiency   There is enough evidence to show sufficient proof of confidence.

The most important guiding principle of APEL is that you have ownership over your own profile. This means that it is up to you to make claims to have your knowledge and skills recognised. So, it is your responsibility to make a claim and support the claim with appropriate evidence. Although you might need support in order to achieve this, it is important to recognise that APEL is concerned with your ability to engage in self-assessment and ultimately take charge of your own learning.

In some cases your profile will be assessed by just one other person. Usually, however, the assessment of your profile will involve at least two other people, and in many cases it will be carried out by an APEL committee. Whoever is involved in the assessment, it will be their job to read the entire profile, weigh up the evidence of learning, and make judgements as to its value. Sometimes this process will be similar to a formal written examination and you will not be involved in the process. More normally, however, the assessment will involve an interview. In the vast majority of cases this interview is conducted in an informal, conversational manner. It is not seen as part of the formal evaluative/assessment process. Rather, interviews are carried out in the spirit of giving positive feedback to aid your future development.

References

FESC (1989) *A Guide to Work-based Learning Terms*, FESC: Bristol

HEQC (1994) *Choosing to Change: The Report of the HEQC CAT Development Project*, HEQC Publications: London

Jessup, G. (1991) *Outcomes: NVQs and the Emerging Model of Education and Training*, Falmer Press: London

Toyne (1979) *Educational Credit Transfer: Feasibility Study*, DES: London

Helping Others to Develop a Profile: The Skills of Facilitation

7

No matter how or when you decide to begin completing your profile, you will expect help from others. Most people find the opportunity of talking through issues and discussing their progress with someone else valuable. Help may come in the form of attending a workshop or short course, or support can usually be harnessed from colleagues, family and friends. However, increasingly people are seeking assistance from those with professional expertise.

In this chapter we will look at some of the specific skills and knowledge you will need in helping someone to complete a profile. We begin by introducing you to some principles about how adults learn and what they bring with them when they embark on a learning programme. We then move on to explore the five key skills of facilitation: enabling; educational counselling; advising; assessing; and informing.

If in an educational situation an adult's experience is ignored, not valued, not made use of, it is not just the experience that is being rejected, it is the person. (Malcolm Knowles, 1984)

This chapter looks at how you can help others to complete their profile. We will explore the specific skills required, as well as some common problems which arise.

In order to fully understand some of these issues, it would be useful for you to understand theories underpinning how adults learn. We begin this chapter, therefore, with an introduction to learning theories which emphasise experience as the source of development. In particular, we look at the importance that the learning process has within the construction of a personal/professional profile, and the relevance of this for professional development.

Learning from experience

The learning which you bring to your working practice has not simply been acquired from formal courses you have attended. Rather, you learn from a broad range of informal learning experiences, such as voluntary activities, leisure pursuits and employment, as well as through family and social situations. So, the learning you use at work is derived from a multiplicity of sources – both at the workplace and outside of work. However, because learning in our culture has so often been associated with formal qualifications, your informal or experiential learning (which often involves considerable effort and expertise) is often disregarded and remains underutilised.

This means that you cannot make assumptions about what you already do or do not know, based simply upon your formal qualifications. Rather, you need to find ways of understanding more about yourself as a learner, and valuing and articulating the extent of your knowledge.

Your interest and willingness to learn will be influenced by many factors, including personal characteristics and motivation; the characteristics and requirements of the particular job you are doing; and the nature and culture of the environment in which you work.

Learning cycle

David Kolb is an American writer who has written extensively on this theme. For Kolb, learning is a cycle (see Figure 5.1 on page 90). We have adapted it as follows:

Figure 7.1 Kolb's learning cycle (adapted)

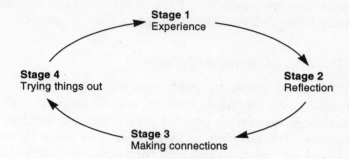

According to this approach, all learning is rooted in experience, but for learning to take place it must actively involve the learner. The emphasis is on learning through discussion, problem-solving and action. What is important in this approach is that the learner comes to internalise what is being learnt in ways which have personal relevance and meaning.

This can be contrasted with traditional approaches to learning, which often promote passive learning gained through the knowledge of an active teacher. This traditional approach is referred to as 'the banking concept' of education; learners are 'filled up with knowledge' which they normally cash in at a later date when they undergo a formal examination process.

Kolb's cycle can be used as a framework to promote learning within the profile process. It brings together theory (reflection/conceptualisation) and practice (experience/testing out), and it can make you aware of your individual approach to learning and learning preference. Understanding *how* you learn is as important as understanding *what* you have learnt, as it helps you to learn more about what motivates or blocks you from learning.

Concrete experience (experience)

In Kolb's learning cycle the learning begins with an experience or event. This might be a specific experience, but it can also include a series of related tasks such as bringing up children or experience of voluntary work. It might also refer to some event you have observed, such as watching a baby being delivered or attending a play or concert.

Reflective observation (reflection)

When you begin to think critically about some of these experiences, you move into the second stage of Kolb's cycle. Although learning is derived from experience, it does not just happen; for learning to take place you need to engage in critical reflection. At this reflective stage, therefore, you begin to identify significant experiences which have the potential to be turned into learning. This involves far more than simply the skills of interpretation. Rather, at its most effective, reflection causes you to ask questions that expand your knowledge and enable you to examine your feelings and values. Through reflection you are able to think carefully about how you approach your work, and thereby extend your professional competence.

One writer who has explored critical reflection in some depth is Jack Mezirow. Mezirow (1983) argues that critical reflection includes the following elements:

- self-examination
- exploring options for new ways of acting
- building competence and self-confidence in new roles
- planning a course of action
- acquiring knowledge and skills necessary for implementing one's plans
- provisional efforts to try new roles and assess feedback
- a reintegration into society on the basis of conditions dictated by the new perspective.

Mezirow calls this process 'perspective transformation'. He argues that perspective transformation provides us:

with the awareness of why we attach the meanings we do to reality, especially to our roles and relationships – meanings often misconstrued out of the uncritically assimilated half-truths of conventional wisdom and power relationships assumed as fixed. (Mezirow, 1983)

Abstract conceptualisation (making connections)

In the third stage, you use reflection to integrate your new experience with past experience. Whereas in the second stage reflection might have lead you to realise that your experience was an isolated example of a general pattern of behaviour, in the third stage you begin to form ideas or theories about what that pattern might be. In this way your learning becomes shaped by past experiences and cultural context, as well as personal values, attitudes and beliefs. This stage is crucial in contributing to individuality and personal identity.

Active experimentation (trying things out)

In the final stage you begin to apply your new ideas to new situations in order to test them out. This stage is particularly important in your professional development, because it provides you with the opportunity to bring together theory and practice. In this way you experiment in ways that might lead to another concrete experience, and so continually move around the learning cycle. You can test new ideas through simulation, role play or in real-life situations. Through role play you can test out theories and ideas without using clients or patients as guinea pigs in the learning process.

Learning style

Experiential approaches to learning recognise that each person has an individual learning style.

As a result of our hereditary equipment, our particular past life experience, and the demands of our present environment, most of us develop learning styles that emphasise some learning abilities over others. Through socialisation experiences, family, school and work, we come to resolve the conflicts between action and reflection between immediate experience and detached analysis in characteristic ways. (Kolb, 1984)

Kolb argues that some people 'excel at assimilating disparate facts into coherent theories, yet these same people may be incapable of, or uninterested in, deducing hypotheses from those theories'. Others may be able to do this, but find it impossible to involve themselves in active experience

Kolb (1984) identifies four commonly occurring learning types:

Convergers These are high scorers on conceptualising ('making connections') and experimentation ('trying things out'). People who exhibit this learning style are said to excel in the application of ideas. They are also characterised as having narrow technical/scientific interests and as being unemotional.

Divergers These are high scorers on concrete experience ('experience') and reflection. People who exhibit this learning style are considered to be imaginative, emotional and interested in people. Their interests are broad and tend to be in the arts.

Assimilators People who fall in this category tend to prefer conceptualisation ('making connections'), together with reflection. They lean toward inductive reasoning, integration of knowledge and the creation of theoretical models. Their social interest is not as strong as that of their divergent colleagues.

Accommodators This learning style is typified by concrete experience ('experience') and experimentation ('testing things out'). People who demonstrate this learning style are good at doing things, trying out new experiences and taking risks. Their approach to problems is said to rely on intuition and trial and error, and is likely to involve other people.

One of the major factors influencing people's preferred learning style is, for Kolb, their current job role. This largely refers to the content of the job, but clearly the relationships they have with their colleagues is also an important factor. So, for example, those people who are working in general management jobs that demand a 'strong orientation to task accomplishment and decision making in uncertain circumstances' require an accommodative learning style. Those people who are working in jobs that demand practical and problem solving skills require a convergent learning style.

Increasingly, as the nature of professional practice changes, you will need to acquire different learning styles in order to accommodate the different requirements of your work.

Assisting others with their profile

Developing a profile is different from almost any other learning activity, in that the curriculum to be studied is not an outside body of knowledge but the learner her/himself. If you are helping someone to construct a profile, therefore, you cannot start by pointing to a pile of books and suggesting that s/he reads these to learn more about a specific topic. Rather, at the outset, you will be helping the profiler to make sense of the knowledge and skills s/he has already learnt and can do, and to make decisions about what the profile should include.

In most learning activities there are two elements. The first is the process through which the learning takes place; this is often referred to as the *how* of learning. The second is the content or substance; this is the *what* of learning. In more traditional approaches to education, the content of learning is largely based on external, existing knowledge available to all. In current (experiential) approaches to professional development, however, greater emphasis is being given to the learning which is intrinsic to the learner, and the process through which that learning occurs.

The skills you need to help others with their profile are almost identical to those used in experiential or open approaches to learning. Professionals who use this type of approach may be known as tutor/counsellor, educational guidance worker, mentor, enabler or educational counsellor. In this book we have chosen to use the term *facilitator*. This is for two reasons. Firstly, in our belief it encapsulates each of the different terms identified above. Secondly, it is the most commonly used and understood term in the field of open and experiential learning.

In order to develop your skills as a facilitator, you need to begin by understanding how adults learn and what they bring with them when they embark on a learning programme. Some learners come with preconceptions about themselves and their ability to learn. Some put up barriers which stop them from learning, whilst others open themselves up to new ideas and concepts. So, you need to understand that each learner is unique, with a wide range of experience, knowledge and skills which they will want to identify and explore.

Blocks to learning

The person you are assisting might simply be completing the profile because it is a requirement by the UKCC and/or they have been told to do so. At worst this might make them hostile to the whole concept; at best they might be prepared only to undertake the bare minimum of work in order to complete the profile.

Some people might feel hesitant about starting because they have not studied for a long time and lack confidence in their knowledge, abilities and experience. Their perception of personal development might be based on their experience of school, where they were perhaps made to feel stupid, or where the information they were learning had little relevance or meaning for them. Certainly, many people who did not perform well at school have been left feeling that education is not for them but for 'clever people'.

Whatever their experience, almost all adults returning to study after a break feel unsure as to their ability to retain knowledge, write for academic purposes, take notes or read effectively. Profiling also raises problems for learners who hold rigid views which have remained unchallenged for a considerable time. Profiling encourages learners to continually question their personal assumptions, values and beliefs about themselves, their profession and the world in which they live.

Challenges to pre-existing knowledge can also present learners with problems. This is particularly true if they are working in a profession where (as in nursing and midwifery) they have traditionally been taught from the received wisdom of others or through direct experience. This is what Rogers (1988) refers to as learning through a 'significant other':

> Any challenge to this learning material, to our existing knowledge implies either a challenge to our significant other (it may be some other respected authority) or a challenge to our self-judgement (we chose to rely on that person, or book, it seemed reasonable at the time) or to both. (Rogers, 1988)

It is also important to remember that most people hold strong beliefs about themselves, their profession and their practice. Through profiling, as people begin to explore and challenge their existing assumptions, they might find a conflict between what they believe about their profession and what they practise; between their personal and professional values and practices. All of this will have implications for how they practise in the future, and it might even lead them to abandon a particular stance or attitude they have upheld in public:

> This will lead some participants to resist learning changes. They will cling to pre-existent knowledge and attitudes and find it hard to assimilate new material or at least not make it harmonize with what is already there. So they adopt mechanisms, most commonly of withdrawal in an attempt to preserve what they already possess. (Rogers, 1988)

Finally, if people are resistant to returning to study, they will identify a host of reasons why their profile will not be successful. Ageing, physical tiredness, declining powers of memory and concentration are all cited as blocks to achievement. Although some might genuinely encounter such problems, research shows that if people are excited, motivated and involved in what they are studying, these factors can usually be overcome. Concentration and memory retention are skills which can be worked on and developed. Again, however, identifying topics which are personally and professionally motivating will improve both of these skills enormously.

Your first task as facilitator, therefore, is to assist the profiler to remove any blocks to learning and, more often than not, to go through a process of unlearning past experiences of education. If the profiler has many barriers to overcome and does not know where to start, you might need to help by finding exercises which will build immediately upon her/his knowledge and abilities. In this way you will be getting rid of any negative self-image and beginning to instil confidence.

Begin by enabling the profiler to identify what these blocks might be. Through the reflective diary, explore these in a positive way and devise personal strategies for overcoming them. The profiler might wish to talk through ideas with you, show you what s/he has written in the diary, or ask your help in developing an action plan for the future. But remember, it is always up to the profiler to determine what help s/he needs from you in order to develop.

Facilitation skills

Facilitating a profile requires a number of complex and interrelated skills. Below we have identified five key skills which we believe all professionals engaged in profile facilitation should possess.

Enabling

At its simplest, enabling means *supporting* the profiler through the development of her/his profile. It involves a number of skills, the most important of which is *listening*. Most learners need someone who will listen carefully and encourage them to articulate their thoughts and ideas. This is called active listening. It means listening carefully to what is being said, whilst at the same time continually challenging the learner to review, analyse and make sense of what s/he is articulating and thinking. Active listening is not easy. Often you will be tempted to interrupt and give the other person your views and ideas on what is being said:

> For some of us, the greatest difficulty of all is to control ourselves, to listen without intervening. Knowing when to shut up has all sorts of aspects: it means knowing that it may be best to keep silent even though there is a pause. It means resisting the temptation to short-circuit the whole process by giving too many lubricating lecturettes, clever, perhaps, and even illuminating, but still not as useful as the students finding their own way in their own time. It means, most of all, shutting up so as to listen better until we hear what is really being said behind often clumsily-chosen words. (Rogers, 1986)

Active listening requires that you stop thinking about yourself and your opinions. Rather, it means genuinely listening to what the profiler is telling you.

Another key enabling skill is to create an environment in which the profiler feels able to speak openly and in confidence about what s/he is thinking and feeling. The profiler should never be encouraged to discuss topics which s/he considers to be private or does not wish to share. The skill lies in enabling the profiler to speak freely about issues which s/he is keen to discuss. So, for example, try to arrange the room in a way which will make the profiler feel relaxed and comfortable, and will create a supportive climate for discussion.

Educational counselling

This refers to helping the profiler to discover, clarify, assess and understand her/his learning in order to plan realistic current and future educational aims and career goals.

Advising

This means helping the profiler to interpret information and to make decisions based on her/his planned learning needs. It might also involve simple advice on where to go for specific information or how to construct a request for a reference letter.

Assessing

Self-assessment is an essential component of profiling. Through careful facilitation you will be enabling the learner to develop confidence in self-assessment and to evaluate the depth and range of her/his learning. Through self-assessment the learner will be much more likely to take control of the profile, to make informed choices about what it should include and to have ownership of it.

Informing

At times it might be appropriate for you to provide information about learning opportunities and professional development policies which might inform the development of the profile. This should be done in a manner which enables the profiler to make her/his own decisions about the specific merits or options from this information.

Taking responsibility

Most people find the prospect of taking responsibility and ownership of their profile daunting. Initially, they argue that they would rather be told what to do. In the early stages, therefore, you might find that the learner is expecting you to tell her/him what to do and how to organise the work. Most people also come to learning with expectations about their tutor. Students often come to learning expecting the facilitator to be both an expert and an authority figure. And, indeed, tutors often feel it is their role to impart knowledge and to tell the students what they should be learning and how this might be achieved. They want to solve all their students problems and provide answers to all their queries.

The worst forms of teaching are often the nicest because they encourage attitudes towards the students and their abilities which, though well-intentioned, are forms of patronage. Inevitably, there are many variants. The most obvious is the man who is over fond of his own voice, who too obviously likes to hear himself speak. A smile appears on his face as he talks, as though he is actually testing the sound of his own rolling periods; you can recognise the element in yourself by the feeling of almost physical pleasure when you are led into that kind of rhetoric. It's like finding you can fly, for a few yards. Those of us who were brought up in the Nonconformist chapel tradition are especially at risk here – the combination of rhetoric, earnestness and the urge towards charismatic relationships is heady. (Richard Hoggart in *Adults Learning*, Jennifer Rogers, 1986)

This approach, then, creates a climate where the student, albeit unintentionally, becomes dependent on the facilitator to make all of the decisions about what and how s/he should be learning. It does little to enable the learner to understand the extent and breadth of her/his learning and to take responsibility for it, all of which is necessary if s/he is to become a more autonomous, thinking professional through a process of self-assessment and profiling:

Life at its best, is a flowing, changing process in which nothing is fixed. Life is richest and most rewarding when it is this flowing process. To experience this is both fascinating and a little frightening. I am at my best when

I can let the flow of my experience carry me, in a direction which appears to be forward, toward goals of which I am but dimly aware. In this stream of my experiencing, and in trying to understand its ever-changing complexity, it should be evident there are no fixed points. There can be no closed system of beliefs, no unchanging set of principles which I hold. Life is guided by a changing understanding of and interpretation of my experience . . . There is no philosophy or belief or set of principle which I could encourage or persuade others to have or hold. I can only try to give others the permission and freedom to develop their own inward freedom and thus their own meaningful interpretation of their own experience. (Rogers, 1971)

This initial stage of helping the profiler to move from being *dependent* on the facilitator, to becoming an *independent* learner, is one of the most valuable aspects of profiling. It is through this process that the profiler should come to understand and appreciate the significance of her/his life experience to date and to develop confidence and self-awareness in her/himself as an individual as well as a professional. In short, if the facilitator listens to and takes seriously what the learner wishes to share, then the learner, in turn, will begin to acknowledge the relevance of her/his ideas and knowledge.

Planning the profile

Developing a profile requires very careful advance planning and preparation. Briefly summarised, there are two planning stages to profiling. In the initial stage, the profiler will be making decisions about whether to develop a profile 'from scratch' or whether to buy one off the shelf. This means s/he will need to think carefully about her/his personal and professional circumstances, and to make decisions about how the materials will be presented and the approach to be adopted. In the second stage the profiler will make decisions about how the profile should be structured, what it should contain, how long it will take to complete and the range and depth of knowledge to be included.

Planning therefore involves identifying the skills, knowledge and attitudes required by both profiler and facilitator, and establishing the learning goals and the individual tasks that need to be completed in order to achieve these objectives. It also involves identifying what resources will be available. These can be human resources, including use of facilitator, family and friends, or they can be physical resources, such as use of library, study area and computer.

You might suggest that the learner spends 2–3 weeks researching what is available by visiting the library, making contact with colleagues and others, and gaining their support.

It is important that during the planning stage the facilitator does not take control. Rather, you should be continually encouraging the learner to take control, identify her/his learning, and make any decisions. This is not as easy as it might sound. Very often as a facilitator it is possible to see all kinds of ways in which your profiler can progress. For example, time and again the profiler will disregard a particular experience as worthless, whereas you might view it as a valuable source of learning. Whilst you might suggest that the profiler 'revisits' the experience to find learning potential, it is always up to the profiler to make connections between learning and experience and decide what s/he wishes to disclose.

It is often the planning stage that is the most difficult. As a facilitator, you need to allow the profiler to take as much time as s/he feels is necessary. However, your task is also to ensure the profile is working within the deadline for completion, and that the profiler has not become 'stuck' and unchallenged. Very often, people beginning a profile find it is the first time they have thought about their past experiences in such a structured and positive way. They find it exciting when long forgotten memories are remembered and they are able to see their life as a learning continuum. If this happens, the learner will fiercely resist any attempt to turn newly acquired learning into a set of competence statements, or translate it into a language which can be immediately assessed. One way to ensure that an effective balance is achieved is through negotiating a learning contract from the outset.

Developing a learning contract

Alan Rogers (1988) argues that in most learning situations a bargain is struck between tutor and student. 'The terms of the bargain may not have been spelled out in full, but the agreement is there none the less.' A learning contract is where the facilitator and the learner work out the details of 'the bargain' in full, and negotiate the terms and conditions. For the profiler, this means asking her/himself a number of fundamental questions:

- Why am I developing a profile?
- Do I understand enough about the profiling process?
- When do I need/wish it to be completed?
- What type of profile do I want?
- What skills have I already got in order to complete it?
- What skills do I need to develop?
- How do I want to use my facilitator?
- What help can I expect from others?

The facilitator needs to ask her/himself:

- How much time am I realistically able to give?
- What skills have I already got in order to facilitate the process?
- What skills do I need to develop?
- Does the profiler's view of the ways in which I am able to help, tally with my own?
- What will my role be in this process?

Setting goals and criteria for success

It is important that you and your profiler openly discuss these questions first, together with any other issues. This should help both of you to clarify the long- and short-term learning goals. So, for example, one long-term goal will be to complete the profile; one short-term goal for achieving this might be to develop written skills to a personal and professional satisfactory standard. The profiler might have more than one long-term goal for the completion of the profile. S/he will usually have several short-term goals.

It is very important that the long- and short-term goals are written down and understood by both of you. Alongside these, the best learning contracts include the criteria for success. Successful criteria for the completion of the profile might include the following.

- I have used it to support an application for a job.
- I have used it to gain academic credit against a course.
- It was constructed, cross-referenced and written to a high personal and professional standard.
- I now understand far more about myself and my professional development needs.

Successful criteria for the completion of written skills might include the following.

- I now have confidence in my writing ability.
- I can construct a sentence using my own words and phrases.
- I now understand the writing process.
- My profile is written clearly, concisely and using my own style.

Drawing up an action plan

The second part of writing a learning contract involves the profiler in working out the actions s/he will take, and the timescale for each, in order to achieve all of her/his goals.

The action plan for developing a personal writing style might include the following statements:

1 Try different writing styles in my reflective diary. See which style I prefer and why.
   Timescale: ongoing throughout the profile process
2 Look at a number of different writing styles used by professionals, including newspapers, journals, reports, novels, etc. Analyse similarities and differences between each; see what I like and dislike.
   Timescale: one month
3 Try approaching the writing of my profile in different ways.
   Timescale: two months
4 Read an article on writing from one of my study skills books.
   Timescale: begin after I have completed actions 2 and 3. Two weeks only
5 Ask family, friends, facilitator to comment on what I have written.
   Timescale: Begin as soon as possible, after two months of commencing my profile

Clarifying the facilitator's role

As the facilitator you will then be in a good position to negotiate *your* terms and conditions. You should discuss the type of support you are able to offer, the amount of time you can give, and the nature of your relationship. An effective profiler–facilitator relationship is one which is an equal partnership. The effectiveness of this equal relationship will affect the quality of the learning experience for the profiler and the outcome of the profile. Your job is primarily to enable the profiler to make the most of the human and physical resources available.

Many profilers might want a more directive relationship, and require you to comment on any written work they have submitted by awarding marks and correcting grammar. It is important when you embark on work, therefore, to explain how you perceive your role and to discuss the need for the profiler to take responsibility for her/his own learning. You might want to indicate that, whilst you are more than happy to comment on work submitted, it is not appropriate for you to correct grammar or award marks in this way. You must carefully explain that, as the facilitator, your role is one of guidance, educational counselling and progress chasing to make sure the profile is completed within the time delineated. But ultimately, it is the profiler who must take ownership of the profile and make decisions as to its development.

This does not mean that you are not able to give your opinion, or to make suggestions as to how the profile can be improved. Rather, it ensures that you are not seen as an expert and authority figure whom the learner can remain dependent upon.

Creating a good learning environment

The facilitator and profiler need to organise the context within which the learning takes place. It means thinking about the environment and the conditions in which both you and the profiler can work effectively. Creating the right learning environment will have an enormous impact on the profiler's motivation, attention and achievement.

Remember that this might be the first time the profiler has been encouraged to talk about such personal issues. However well the profiler knows you, s/he will probably feel nervous or apprehensive about doing so. Clearly, then, it is important to create an atmosphere which feels 'safe' and inviting.

In addition, the profiler will not always want to meet with you alone. Sometimes, s/he will wish to meet with peers, colleagues, friends and others to share issues and brainstorm ideas. Will you be able to find suitable accommodation for small group work? If not, can your profiler suggest an appropriate place in which to meet?

David Boud *et al* (1985) suggest that learners need *freedom to learn*. They need to be free from the pressures of their everyday lives in order to think and reflect. This means that people need to allow themselves space and time to study, but many feel guilty about taking time out to learn. Try and encourage your profiler not to feel guilty. Build sufficient time into your meetings for her/him to block out all the external factors s/he will bring into the room. Find ways of enabling her/him to throw out the 'daily baggage' for a short time.

Establishing ground rules

Creating the appropriate conditions in which to learn also means that both of you need to establish the ground rules within which you can both work. Within a conventionally taught course, the ground rules are much more clear. Each college has a mission statement and prospectus which makes clear to the student what resources are available and what are not. This will include use of computer and library facilities, as well as attendance at lectures and seminars and tutor allocation and role.

The learning contract is an excellent place for you both to establish ground rules. The profiler will be able to state what s/he wants to achieve and how s/he wishes to achieve it. This in turn means that the profiler is acknowledging responsibility for her/his own learning.

As facilitator, you must make your role equally clear. This means establishing when you are available and, equally, when you are not. You should also acknowledge that in this role you are not a counsellor. This is important. Sometimes, when the profiler is discussing personal aspects of her/his life, this might throw up a specific, emotionally charged experience which s/he has not thought about or confronted before. In this situation the profiler might well need to find someone to talk it through and help her/him to understand or come to terms with it. These kinds of skills are not skills for the facilitator. Rather, you need to point the profiler in the direction of someone who is professionally trained to help.

In addition, you need to clarify any expectations you might have from your profiler. So, for example, you might wish to establish rules about ensuring you both keep to agreed starting and ending times of meetings. Working within an agreed time framework will help to ensure the discussion is more focused and achieves the objectives your profiler has set.

Progress chasing

Perhaps the most important element of facilitation lies in challenging the profiler to move through the different stages of development to completion. This is not as easy as it sounds. Most people find that, once they have overcome their initial fears, thinking about their past experience is fascinating and of great interest. They enjoy the process of reflection and of exploring their personal and professional lives. They find it difficult to move into *analysing* what they have learnt from their experience and *documenting* this in a way which makes sense and can be assessed by others.

The learning contract, again, will form a sound framework from which you and the profiler can review progress. There may be legitimate reasons why the profiler is not progressing as quickly as anticipated. The learning contract should be continually renegotiated and new deadlines set. However, your job is to enable the profiler to be honest as to the reasons for any delay, and to identify where there are blocks to progress and how these might be overcome.

Evaluation

Whether you are facilitating or learning, you need to find ways of working out how effective you have been. Evaluation is simply a process of enabling you to do so. Evaluation should enable you to think about your facilitation skills, identify your weaknesses and map out ways of building upon your strengths. Evaluation is an essential component of the learning process.

There are two forms of evaluation, **formative** and **summative**. Formative evaluation is the ongoing continuous evaluation that goes on throughout the learning process. Summative evaluation is that which takes place when the profile has been finally completed. In reality, of course, both feed into each other. The learner should be actively involved in both forms of evaluation. This is just as true when you are evaluating your facilitation skills. The profiler should be continually giving feedback as to whether you are effectively supporting her/his learning needs.

At the heart of this process are the questions that both facilitator and profiler must address:

- To what extent is the profiler developing and engaging in the profiling process?
- What is the quality and level of her/his development?
- How much of what is incorporated into the profile is owned and understood by the profiler?
- How motivated is the profiler to develop?

Questions for you to ask, therefore, are more to do with how well the learner is developing than how well you are performing as a facilitator.

In this chapter we have highlighted some of the key issues you need to address in facilitating the profiling process. If you would like to explore the subject in more depth there are many books currently available. You will find some suggested reading in the Annotated Bibliography.

References

Boud, D., Keogh, R. and Walker, R. (1985) *Reflection: Turning Experience into Learning*, Kogan Page: London

Knowles, M. (1984) *Andragogy-in-action*, Jossey Bass: San Francisco

Kolb, D. (1984) *Experiential Learning: Experience as the Source of Learning and Development*, Prentice Hall: New Jersey

Mezirow, J. (1983) 'A Critical Theory of Adult Learning and Education', in M. Tight (ed) *Adult Learning and Education*, Croom Helm: Kent

Rogers, A. (1988) *Teaching Adults*, OU Press: Milton Keynes

Rogers, C. (1971) *On Becoming a Person: A Therapist's View of Psychotherapy*, Redwood Press: London

Rogers, J. (1986) *Adults Learning* (2nd edn), OU Press: Milton Keynes

Epilogue

Through writing this book we found we had raised as many questions as we had tried to answer. We found ourselves returning to a number of stubborn issues that could not be easily answered, but we felt needed to be addressed if profiling is to have any real relevance within nursing and midwifery. These issues are about confidentiality, cost effectiveness, assessment criteria, and how profiles fit into a wider agenda currently running in the health service. Because of this, we decided to record a conversation between ourselves about some of these issues. This conversation is our contribution to the debate and we hope it will inspire you to carry it on in your own field.

Where is the introduction of profiling taking nursing and midwifery?

Liz: Profiles are relatively new in nursing and midwifery and the professions are beginning to embrace the concepts fairly well. The introduction of profiles to get educational credit in nursing and midwifery was the first time experience, knowledge and skills had been valued in that way. Before then many nurses and midwives felt that their previous experience was not always worthwhile unless they had a qualification to go with it.

As I hope we have shown in the book, if you take the

broader view of the profiling process it can be a great way of increasing your self-esteem and confidence, because you can use it to gain a real sense of yourself and your strengths and weaknesses. If the use of profiling becomes as widespread as it could, then the combined effect of all that work can be very positive for the profession as a whole. It will take nurses and midwives to a point where they feel more confident about themselves and the skills and knowledge they have. There is the potential for profiling to improve practice by encouraging nurses and midwives to reflect on their practice. It will also help them to identify and fulfil their continuing development needs.

Is profiling here to stay?

Liz: I believe so, though its use will change and evolve over time. One of the most interesting things about profiling in nursing and midwifery is the extent to which it has both professional and political clout behind it. In my 25 years' experience in the profession, I would say it is quite unusual to have the combination of professional and political will behind an initiative. I am sure it will succeed. It cannot be a '10-minute wonder' because, for one thing, it will take until 2001 for everyone on the register to be incorporated into the use of profiles to re-register. What will happen after that we can only speculate about.

Where is the introduction of personal profiling taking other professional groups?

Cathy: From the mid 1980s profiles were signalled as one of the most powerful means through which learning, in its broadest sense, could be assessed and accredited by higher education. In this sense it was seen as making an important contribution to the changing face of higher education, supporting many initiatives associated with flexible, experiential and open learning. But what has its effect been on professional groups outside nursing and midwifery?

There are a number of professions outside of nursing and midwifery that have effectively adopted some of the principles associated with profiling. Social work, for example, was one of the first professions to have foreseen its importance and relevance. However, commerce and industry have also effectively taken the concept of profiling into the workforce, albeit not requiring people to complete a personal profile. The philosophy underpinning profiling is used within management training and education. Much of the management literature is now littered with references to experiential learning, reflective practice, learning contracts and self-evaluation. These ideas have largely been taken from what could loosely be termed the 'experiential' or 'profiling' movement, and have been very successful. So, increasingly, organisations are using profiles with their middle and senior management posts.

What is particularly exciting about how profiling has been developed within nursing is that it has been targeted for use by staff at all levels. Moreover, it is concerned with linking theory with practice, and creating what Schon refers to as reflection-in-action. In nursing, profiling is concerned with clinical as well as generic management processes, both of which are important to the nurse of the future.

Will profiling be continued to be emphasised over the next ten years, both within and outside of nursing and midwifery?

Liz: As I've said before, profiling will not be a '10-minute wonder'. I think it is really impressive that nurses and midwives have started initiatives such as clinical supervision, profiling and reflective practice, and they are being supported not only by the academics within the profession and the writers who try to convince others, but by the statutory bodies and by Government (in the sense that it supports the policies of the statutory bodies). This is quite a unique situation. Now profiling is in the statute, it will take the UKCC until 2001 to actually implement. What happens after that we will have to wait and see. I believe profiling will go from strength to strength.

Outside of nursing and midwifery it seems that current trends, like life-long learning, experiential and open learning, and reflective practice, have profiling at their core. We can even see evidence of profiling in secondary school education, with pupils being required to complete records of achievement. These initiatives all complement each other, and by building up a web of commonality profiling gains a certain strength that perhaps other initiatives in the past have not had.

Cathy: Nurses and midwives are increasingly required to fund their own continuing education and development. Clearly this makes a difference to the kind of education and training they are able to undertake. This, coupled with the fact that many nurses and midwives are unable to negotiate study leave, makes profiling a very popular option. Firstly, as we have stated throughout this book, it is a process which can cost very little money, depending on what the profile is being used for. It is only when people decide to have their profile assessed against an academic course and to gain credit, that there is a cost attached. Secondly, the profile process should help people to identify realistic future educational and career-related goals. In this way they don't have to waste time and money on courses which have no benefit.

Liz: Employers are now demanding much more of higher education; they want to make sure that people leaving programmes are equipped with the knowledge and skills relevant to the industry or profession the person is entering. This is the 'fitness for purpose' idea. Employers also want the workforce to be creative, flexible and adaptable to change.

Cathy: Because of the initiative such as the Patient's Charter, nurses and midwives are more than ever having to critically reflect upon their practice. If a particular treatment is not provided, or not provided to the patient's satisfaction, in theory he or she has the opportunity to complain. Health care professionals, therefore, need to be able to justify and defend their actions.

What is the future of profiling in nursing and midwifery?

Liz: I believe there is the potential for profiling to go a really long way. At one level there is a minimalist approach where everyone will just do what the UKCC requires and this will be a way of people recording their learning through self-assessment. However, there is the potential for profiles to do much more than that. For a while we are likely to have two or three parallel processes going on where people are either just getting their heads down to fulfil UKCC requirements, or they will be challenged more and more to think about profiling in its widest sense. Hopefully nurses and midwives will begin to understand how profiles can be used in a much greater way than the UKCC demands. This will be positive for nursing and midwifery; if people can begin to build up skills to enable them to use the profile in a multitude of ways, the benefits, in terms of understanding their own skills, abilities and worth, will be incredibly positive for the profession.

I believe that the collective psychology of the nursing and midwifery profession shows you that it has quite a low self-esteem. I believe the widespread use of profiles can make a difference to this.

What impact will profiles have on the knowledge base of nursing and midwifery?

Liz: We already gain our nursing and midwifery knowledge from a number of sources, such as our own practice and the theories and research of other people, but there is a rich source of knowledge that will be contained in the reflective writings within profiles. Where people are recording what they have learnt from their practice, those points of learning may well be generally applicable to other professionals dealing with similar problems. Unfortunately people tend to keep these things to themselves, but if we can learn to trust and share those bits of our individual knowledge with others, we can collectively build up another source of knowledge, which at the moment is inaccessible.

As a non-nurse, how do you think the nursing and midwifery profession has dealt with the profiling issue?

Cathy: I can think of no other profession which has had the confidence or foresight to implement the concepts of reflective practice and profiling across the whole of its workforce. Outside of nursing and midwifery the main push for profiling has come from further and higher education, through reforms in qualifications and particularly through the assessment and accreditation of prior experiential learning. Within nursing and midwifery, profiling has come from a very different base. The profession has taken on profiling in order to change the role of the nurse and midwife, and to contribute to more effective patient care. Nursing and midwifery as a profession can only be applauded and supported for this effort.

How easy is it for nurses and midwives to discuss their practice critically in a small group setting such as a clinical supervision group?

Liz: There are difficulties. Some groups of staff have set themselves up because they see the benefit in sharing practice and discussing the issues that are raised in a supportive way. This creates difficulties because nursing and midwifery is not generally used to this. Sharing reflective or profiling practices is a concept which is being introduced on top of a history of nurses and midwives not really being encouraged to share what they do – if they are encouraged to share, it is often used to criticise rather than in a developmental way. For example, it would be useful to use a profile as part of an annual performance review, but a lot of nurses and midwives have a sceptical view of individual performance review. They do not see it as a way of getting feedback on what they have achieved, or helping them to know where they are going in the future. It is often used as a way of criticising, rather than encouraging.

This history does not help when you ask groups of people to get together in order to work out the future of their practice. People have concerns about confidentiality, about how the information is going to be used, and we discuss these issues in the book. These problems are not peculiar to profiling, they also occur in the implementation of clinical supervision.

Is there anything we can do about this?

Liz: Yes. Trust will have to be built up over a period of time with each group and facilitator. This will happen if we start to encourage sharing habits in a safe environment in initial, pre-qualifying programmes. It is very difficult to find ways of rewarding the work people put into profiles. Even within educational programmes it is difficult to find adequate ways of assessing them. It is interesting that performance-related pay has often been rejected by the nursing and midwifery profession. There are probably more fears than positive feelings about performance being attached to reward. Profiling gets caught up in all these feelings too.

Cathy: If everyone knew how to assess and facilitate the whole profiling process and was sympathetic to the philosophy underpinning the reflective practice movement, then profiling could be really powerful.

Liz: The best appraisal interviews have almost been like profiling interviews. Managers who have handled this process well, even if the member of staff maybe has not achieved as much as s/he or the manager wanted, come out of that process feeling very positive about the future.

Experience has been gained in assessing profiles for educational purposes, but how can this be done more effectively by managers and employers?

Cathy: There is a problem because most managers do not know how to assess profiles – they do not know how to read them. I have some sympathy with this, because the assessment of a profile is difficult and requires a number of complex skills. Part of the problem for managers is that, whilst they might understand the philosophy of profiling, in the main they do not know enough about the profile process. If they don't understand how the profile 'works', they will not be able to assess one.

Also, if profiles are going to be used for access to jobs and career opportunities, it will require managers to think more carefully about what they want people to do in their jobs. Job descriptions are often written without thinking about the specific knowledge, skills and qualities which will be required to complete specific tasks.

Managers need to develop a set of criteria which matches up to job specifications. In this way, the use of profiles in the job application process becomes the dual responsibility of the manager and the applicant. The manager needs to make quite clear what a specific job will entail, and the criteria through which s/he will be assessing an applicant's ability to carry out the job. It is then the applicant's responsibility to demonstrate skills and knowledge against these criteria.

What do we see when we both look at the profiles in a global context?

Liz: I find it exciting that British nursing and midwifery is leading the world in the way we are approaching the use of profiles. We have an example in the first chapter from Ontario, Canada, where they were looking to see how they could use profiles in a new quality assurance programme. Initially they looked to the USA, their immediate neighbour, to see what was happening. They did not find what they wanted there and came to Britain; they found what they needed here and have used it in their strategy.

Cathy: I agree, it is exciting. The concept of profiles has largely been derived from America, where profiling has been part of higher education for a long time. However, I believe that we have moved far beyond what is happening in the American context. What we have in Britain is a very unique form of profiling, both within and outside of nursing. This is because we have taken key adult education principles about personal empowerment and applied these to the profile process. What is interesting is the extent to which other countries have looked at what is happening in Britain and are trying to develop similar approaches. So, there are lots of ways in which we are influencing what is happening in other nursing contexts. I think we can say that not only are we leading the field in this country, we are also influencing what is happening in professional development across the world.

Liz: I think we need to make sure that this is known. It is important that people in this country who are leading projects to implement profiling actually make that known – nationally, of course, but also internationally. We should take opportunities to go to conferences and write papers. It is nice to be able to say that British nursing and midwifery is leading the way.

Cathy: This is something to be proud of. If what we believe about the benefits of profiling to the profession holds true, then the use of profiles should have tremendously positive effects on nursing and midwifery over the next ten years.

Liz: It probably would have been much easier for the UKCC to have gone along the route that a lot of other countries have taken – credited programme systems – to ensure that nurses and midwives were fit to re-register. One of the reasons that the Ontario development occurred was that they were quite dissatisfied with what they were seeing in Canada and the rest of North America, and wanted to find some new way to look at the issue. Here we have a new way which they felt was attractive. I think it is very positive.

Cathy: Nursing and midwifery has been successful in its implementation of profiling because the profession, as a whole, began by agreeing the philosophy upon which profiling rests, and then it worked out how this philosophy could be implemented in practice.

Profiles can be done in a number of different ways for different reasons. What single factor would we wish to retain and embed into any future developments of professional profiles for nurses and midwives?

Liz: For me it is the way profiles can give you feedback on what you have been doing. Over a period of time, building up information in a profile gives you a map of your life, and certainly your professional life, that you can look back on at any time. I call this a professional life map. We rarely get the opportunity to look back on our achievements in this way. It can be a tremendously rewarding experience if we give ourselves an opportunity to look back on what we have done. It shows you what you have learnt from the past and gives you a platform for the future – a real sense of what you have achieved and what you have learnt from your achievements. This is a really important message about profiles that I would want to give. They give you a building block, both for your future career and professional development. Often the process of writing about our experiences in the profile – actually getting them out of your head and putting them on paper – is a chance for people to get insights into what they have learnt which they do not get from anywhere else. Those insights can be such gifts for the future.

Cathy: When Sir Christopher Ball was at the RSA and involved with its Education for Capability initiative, he said that one characteristic of being human is the desire to learn, and the more we learn the more we become human in some way.

What has always interested me about professional education is that it can often be very flat and dry. By that I mean that people do not approach it with the same level of enthusiasm they approach other courses, hobbies and activities. What is exciting about profiling is that it is eclectic and values learning wherever it happens. People can bring all of their interests, values and passions to their professional development through this process.

I have seen people really excited and passionate about doing their profiles, in the same way as I have seen them excited about reading a novel or painting a picture. For me, what I want to hold good is an approach to professional development that makes people passionate about seeking knowledge, about finding out about themselves and about going out into the world and learning new things. I want nurses and midwives to experience the excitement and commitment to knowledge which makes professional learning desirable, and thereby much more human.

Annotated Bibliography

Profiling documents and texts

Brown, R. A. (1995) *Portfolio Development and Profiling for Nurses* **(2nd edn)**, Central Health Studies Series No. 3. (series editor, John Tingle), Lancaster: Quay Publishing
This updated publication offers a well-structured guide to developing your profile, including the collection of material for specific purposes. It provides a good, easy-to-read introduction to the subject.

Cambridge Professional Profile. PO Box 56, Oldham OL2 5NZ
This document is divided into four sections: personal details; professional record; personal development planning; and miscellaneous types of evidence with preprinted sheets on which to write. The profile provides little more than a framework within which to develop your own document. There are very few activities to help develop your thinking and skills.

Churchill Livingstone Professional Portfolio for Nurses, Midwives and Health Visitors **(1993)**, Churchill Livingstone: Edinburgh
Designed with the user in mind, this personal portfolio offers a lucid and concise framework within which to build a personalised account of your career: past, present and future.

157

The binder is divided into two distinct parts, with labelled dividers for the different sections. Part A focuses on profiles, general and professional education, professional employment and professional development. It provides you with a place to record your personal details, under pre-printed headings, associated with the above. It will be particularly useful in relation to developing your curriculum vitae (CV), applying for a new post, and seeking accreditation of prior learning. Part B helps you to focus on your current and future development, addressing the areas of goal planning and review, critical incident analysis, development of action plans, continuing education activities, and CV writing. This will be particularly useful in relation to performance review, preparation of development plans, and documenting evidence for UKCC purposes.

Developing Your Personal Professional Portfolio(1995), Churchill Livingstone: Edinburgh
This is a free-standing module from the *Professional Development for Quality Care* series, written specifically for practising nurses, midwives and health visitors. This extremely interactive workbook, with a supplementary reader of journal articles, encourages practitioners to explore the issues raised within the text and relate them to their own areas of practice. It takes a broad-based approach to developing your portfolio and incorporates, amongst other issues, sections on collecting evidence; improving learning skills; the art of making connections; exploring your life experience; exploring your work experience; and getting credit for academic, management and professional purposes. Areas of interest can be studied further by using the annotated reading list.

English National Board (1991) *Professional Portfolio*, ENB Publications: London
This document is an essential component for those practitioners who are indexed for the Higher Award, although any practitioner can purchase and use it. The binder contains a series of useful summary cards that provide a brief

explanation of important areas, including the ten key charac-teristics, credit accumulation and transfer, and pathways through the framework. There are discrete sections with organised headings, followed by a series of blank pages. There is an underpinning emphasis that encourages you to reflect on your past, present and planned future activities.

Macmillan Open Learning (1994) *Profile Pack*, Macmillan Magazines: London

The design of this pack is based on an open learning package. You are encouraged to participate in, and reflect upon, a variety of activities interspersed throughout the text. The pack provides a comprehensive document that can be used for both public and private purposes. The first part of the profile has been created to enable you to review your current situation, both personally and professionally, utilising a variety of activities. The second part focuses on pro-fessional diary keeping. The third part concentrates on the 'private' record where sensitive information can be stored. The emphasis of this profile is on thinking about both your personal and professional lives. It includes a good supply of carbonised goal and action plan record sheets.

Professional Nurse Personal Professional Profile. Mosby

This document is divided into three parts: making a rational career plan; planning your continuing education; and preparing your CV. Printed fact sheets are provided for recording the details of your career and participation in continuing education activities (refill packs can be bought separately). Interactive activities called Action Points are included, which help you to develop insights into yourself and your development needs. Target lists for action planning and review are also included at regular intervals throughout the profile.

Student Profile. Mosby

This profile is designed specifically for the student health care professional. It is interactive, with two types of self-completion activity. Fact sheets and Action Points are included, along the lines of the *Professional Nurse Personal Professional Profile*. There are four parts: part 1 provides the opportunity to develop a detailed record of progress through the course; part 2 encourages you to take stock of the wider aspects of development, including non-work activities; part 3 concentrates on the skills you will need to succeed as a student; and part 4 focuses on career planning and the identification of career opportunities.

Study skills

Northedge, A. (1990) *The Good Study Guide*, OU Press: Milton Keynes

This book is good for students who are re-entering formal learning after a long break and experienced students who need to develop one or more aspects of their study technique. The book is interactive, with activity breaks at regular intervals. Key point summaries are also provided (in a different colour) to help you to focus your mind on your specific learning. In addition to the issues covered in most study skills guides, this book looks at handling numbers confidently. It is designed to meet the needs of social science and humanities students, including adults studying part-time.

Rowntree, D. (1988) *Learn How to Study* (3rd edn), Warner: London

This book has been a bestseller since 1970. It has been updated to include the latest research findings related to effective study. It introduces the idea of reflection in the preface. The basic philosophy appears to be the empowerment of students by encouraging the examination of a range of approaches to study, thereby enabling them to utilise the most appropriate technique based upon their personal preference and the purpose of their study. The book is extremely easy to read, with many interactive activities interspersed throughout the theoretical text.

Rowntree, D. (1993) *Teach Yourself with Open Learning* **(2nd edn)**, Kogan Page: London

This lively and engaging book helps learners to make the most of what is available for them in learning. Although the focus is on open learning, the approach is relevant to profile development and reflective practice. The book provides the opportunity to 'dip in' as required and has bold headings and chapter objectives that help you to decide what you want to read. The activities, interspersed throughout the book, provide you with adequate space to note your thoughts. Follow-up activities, which often rely upon interaction with others, provide the opportunity to apply the theory to your practice. Each chapter culminates in a 'reflective activity' that encourages you to sit down and think about your learning.

Career development

Bolles, R. (1996) *What Colour is Your Parachute?* Ten Speed Press: Enfield, Middlesex

This book, which is updated annually, is the UK edition of the best-selling US guide to self-analysis and pro-active jobhunting. The British edition comprises the US text with its variety of interactive exercises. The 'pink pages' at the back, which provide a resource directory, is unfortunately heavily influenced by availability within the US. However, the overall system is well tried and tested.

Covey, R. (1989) *The 7 Habits of Highly Effective People*, Simon and Schuster: East Roseville, New South Wales, Australia

This best-selling book helps you to solve both personal and professional problems by adopting a holistic, integrated and principle-centred approach. It provides many anecdotes and insights into 'effectiveness'. Covey presents a programmed journey for living, with the emphasis on integrity, fairness, honesty and adaptability to change. He asserts that these are essential features if you are to take advantage of the opportunities that change creates. The book is enhanced by the Application Suggestions which are included at the end of each chapter.

Hopson, B. and Scally, M. (1991) *Build Your Own Rainbow: A Workbook for Career and Life Management*, Mercury: London

This interactive and easy-to-use workbook comprises a number of exercises designed to help you analyse and develop your personal skills, talents and aspirations. It provides the key to a number of essential career development skills, including self-awareness, learning from experience, research skills, goal setting and action planning, decision making and communicating. The exercises in the book encourage you to discover what is important to you about your work, interests and transferable skills. You will be helped to set personal career objectives and make action plans to enable you to take more control of yourself and your life.

Peddlar, M. and Boydell, T. (1989) *Managing Yourself,* Harper Collins: London

This is one of the early books of the *Successful Manager* series. This practical guide contains case studies and useful activities that are designed to help you enhance your practice of self-management, with a view to improving your life and performance at work and elsewhere. The book provides a logical approach, introducing themes, developing them further, and offering an opportunity for in-depth analysis. You are encouraged to use the analysis to make decisions and action plan your life, implement your plan and review the outcomes of your action. This process is achieved in a variety of ways, including questionnaires, case studies to promote thinking, and exercises to improve self-management. The final chapter is blank – apart from the heading – as it is for you to develop your personal plan.

Rouillard, L. (1993) *Goals and Goal Setting*, Kogan Page: London

The authors consider that this book is unlike many on the

subject. It is 'designed to be read with a pencil', with an abundance of activities, exercises, case studies and assessments that require learner participation. The object of the book is to enhance understanding and valuing of personal goals and goal setting. It provides a good, basic introduction to the level of achievement which goal setting can accomplish. The book could be used in many ways, including individual study, workshops and seminars, and informal study groups.

Wright, B. (1992) *Which Way Now? How to Plan and Develop a Successful Career*, Piatkus: London

This book claims to be a self-investor's guide to life, work and career – full of good sense, help and pragmatism. It suggests ways in which you can be in control of your future; shows how to set short- and long-term goals; demonstrates how to match your skills and values with the right jobs; and shows how to use creative thinking to develop your career. Phase 1 explores aspects of self-knowledge. Phase 2 focuses on exploring your options, including going it alone. Phase 3 concentrates on action planning and basic communication skills, personal presentation and written communication skills. Phase 4 concludes with career monitoring and career maintenance.

Ways of learning

Boud, D., Cohen, R. and Walker, D. (eds) (1993) *Using Experience for Learning*, SRHE/OU Press: Buckingham

This book addresses the struggle of trying to make sense of learning from experience. It explores concepts such as: What are the key ideas that underpin 'learning from experience'? How do we learn from experience? How does context and purpose influence learning? How does experience impact on individual and group learning? How can we help others to learn from their experience? This book addresses the use of experiential learning in the contexts of informal and formal learning. It does not offer simple strategies of how to make it work, but explores the underpinning philosophy of experiential learning.

Boud, D. and Griffin V. (1989) *Appreciating Adults' Learning: From the Learner's Perspective*, Kogan Page: London

The majority of books about how people learn are written from the teacher's or psychologist's perspective. In contrast, this book is written from the learner's perspective, focusing on issues that are important to learners and how they feel about them. The book is enhanced further by the inclusion of learning from work and general experience.

Boud, D., Keogh, R. and Walker, D. (1985) *Reflection: Turning Experience into Learning*, Kogan Page: London

This book synthesises the many theoretical insights, from across a variety of fields, about the potential of reflection. Furthermore, these insights are illuminated with recent practical examples. Thus, the relation of theory to practice (and vice versa) is well illustrated. The book contains an examination of the nature of reflection and its role in the learning process. It focuses on the place of writing, discussion and conversation in reflection.

Brookfield, D. (1987) *Developing Critical Thinkers: Challenging Adults to Explore Alternative Ways of Thinking and Acting*, OU Press: Milton Keynes

This book aims to introduce readers to critical thinking. The central theme is the need to make the connection between the reader's private life and the broader social forces. It examines the methods that can be used by those seeking to introduce the concept of critical thinking to others. It also explores the opportunities for developing critical thinking in four specific areas: intimate relationships; workplace; political involvement; and the mass media. The book is divided into three sections: the concept of critical thinking; helping people to become critical thinkers; and opportunities for developing critical thinking in specific contexts. The book is well illustrated with case studies and exercises, and also includes an extensive reference list.

Downs, S. (1995) *Learning at Work,* Kogan Page: London
This lively, easy-to-use book is designed to help manager, trainer and learner to recognise and overcome obstacles to learning. It provides a practical guide to understanding and practising the concepts that help people learn. The book is interspersed throughout with cartoons and checklists to amplify its message. It also points out the myths, pitfalls and blockages that stand in the way of successful learning. The book is divided into seven sections: sections 1 and 2 explore beliefs about learning; section 3 concentrates upon designing training material for learning; section 4 focuses on developing training material to develop understanding; section 5 discusses developing learning through group involvement; section 6 provides an example of a workshop ('Working safely in times of change'); and section 7 suggests some criteria to use when reviewing training materials.

Evans, N. (1994) *Experiential Learning for All,* Cassel Education: Guildford and Kings Lynn
This book offers a snapshot portrayal of experiential learning in the various contexts in which it has developed over the last decade. Each chapter provides a different focus, and in doing so draws on the experience of practitioners from many fields of education. Assessment of prior experiential learning is defined and considered in the contexts of higher education, further education, adult education, the professions, teacher education, employment and unemployment, assessment, staff development and, finally, international developments. The concluding chapter projects the future of the assessment of experiential learning.

Marshall, L. and Rowland, F. (1993) *A Guide to Learning Independently* **(2nd edn),** OU Press: Milton Keynes
This book offers a comprehensive range of techniques to help you succeed in education. It emphasises the importance

of identifying your own learning needs and the techniques that best suit you. This latest edition includes new study techniques and advice based on current learning theory and research. Updated topics include correct referencing and the use of computers in tasks such as essay writing. The diverse cultural background of students is acknowledged. This is a book for a wide range of students and teachers, engaged in both practical and theoretical courses and in science and humanities. Although there is a degree of interactivity, it is not as obvious as for many other study skills workbooks.

McNiff, J. (1993) *Teaching as Learning: An Action Research Approach*, Routledge: London

This book presents the author's account of her own work and professional development. The study is based on the hypothesis that educational knowledge is created by individuals at work, rather than by researchers in institutions of higher education. The aim of this book is to encourage practitioners to make sense of their own practice, while evaluating the contributions of other thinkers to this understanding. This fascinating and personal book works with case studies of actual practice. The author uses the familiar action research paradigm of identifying a problem; imagining, implementing and evaluating a solution; and modifying practice in the light of that evaluation. She gives practical advice that will aid the professional development of the researcher and practitioner alike. She concludes that the best teaching is done by those who want to learn and can show others how to be open to their own processes in self-development.

Open University (1992) *Accrediting Prior Learning: A Training Pack for Advisors and Assessors*, OU Press: Milton Keynes

This extensive learning pack will assist those professionals wishing to develop their skills in the management of accreditation of prior experiential learning (APEL). It covers a variety of topics, including facilitating APEL; supporting and guiding candidates; what constitutes evidence; assessing a claim for learning from experience; negotiating; and action plans.

Palmer, A., Burns, S. and Bulman, C. (eds) (1994) *Reflective Practice in Nursing: The Growth of the Professional Practitioner,* Blackwell Scientific: London

This book provides an easy-to-read resource for nurse practitioners and educationalists who wish to explore the area of reflective practice in nursing. Its contributors come from a wide range of backgrounds, but are all actively engaged in the development of reflective practice. The book takes you through the various stages of reflection and encourages you to to make more sense of clinical practice. There is no requirement to read the book from cover to cover, as its style enables you to dip into the aspect in which you are most interested. This aspect might be the nature and theories of reflective learning, the facilitation and assessment of reflective learning, or your personal experience, for example.

Weil, S. and McGill, I. (eds) (1989) *Making Sense of Experiential Learning,* SHRE/OU Press: London

This book explores the multiplicity of meanings and practices associated with experiential learning in an international context. The editors have identified four discrete perspectives from amongst the contributors. These different perspectives are identified as 'villages', which contribute towards the 'global village'. The book illustrates the complexities of experiential learning and challenges readers to use the benefits of experiential learning in their own lives.

Whittaker, P. (1995) *Managing to Learn,* Cassell: London

This readable, well-researched book is one of the Cassell series of *Pastoral Care and Personal and Social Education.* The premise for the book is that the ability to facilitate learning is one of the most awesome tasks that a teacher confronts. It helps teachers to organise learning in such a way that individual student's potential is released and capitalised upon, whilst societal needs are also met. The author's main theme is that the student requires instruction for knowledge and practice, alongside the opportunity to develop the skills to reflect deliberately upon the process of learning itself. Although this book is apparently written for school teachers, the content is applicable to adult education. Section 1 – Learners and Learning – draws on the work of Knowles, Freire and Boud and Walker, for example. Section 2 – Teachers and Teaching – reviews the role of the teacher as both a manager and a leader, providing some frameworks to work within. Section 3 – Classrooms and Schools – is applicable to any learning organisation. Section 4 – The A–Z of Learning – provides definitive paragraphs based around terminology on topics such as accountability, beliefs, communication and emotion.

Index

169